Pediatric Dentistry - A Comprehensive Guide

Edited by Mandeep Singh Virdi

Published in London, United Kingdom

Pediatric Dentistry - A Comprehensive Guide
http://dx.doi.org/10.5772/intechopen.102168
Edited by Mandeep Singh Virdi

Contributors
Krishna Patil, Rucha Davalbhakta, Smita Patil, Sujatha P, Chetana Jagtap, Buneet Kaur, Siddhrath Shinde, Ichiro Nakajima, Ryosuke Koushi, Atsushi Uchida, Taketo Yamaguchi, Dinorah Munira Hernández-Santos, Irma Fabiola Díaz-García, Ana Bertha Olmedo-Sánchez, Luz Elena Nápoles-Salas, Kempaiah Siddaiah Madhusudhan, M.R. Pallavi, Shubha Joshi, Pronob Sanyal, Jyotsna Arun Patil

First published in London, United Kingdom, 2023 by IntechOpen
IntechOpen is the global imprint of INTECHOPEN LIMITED, registered in England and Wales, registration number: 11086078, 5 Princes Gate Court, London, SW7 2QJ, United Kingdom

British Library Cataloguing-in-Publication Data
A catalogue record for this book is available from the British Library

Additional hard and PDF copies can be obtained from orders@intechopen.com

Pediatric Dentistry - A Comprehensive Guide
Edited by Mandeep Singh Virdi
p. cm.
Print ISBN 978-1-80355-966-7
Online ISBN 978-1-80355-967-4
eBook (PDF) ISBN 978-1-80355-968-1

Meet the editor

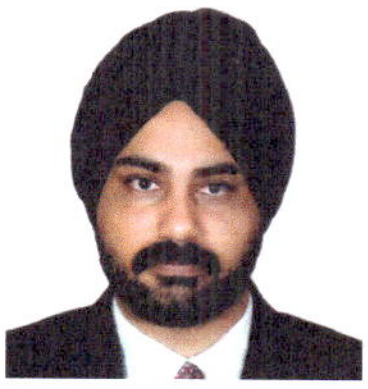

Dr. Mandeep Singh Virdi has an MDS in Pediatric Dentistry and is a highly accomplished and respected pediatric dentist in Delhi, India. His extensive training and experience have equipped him with the knowledge and skills to provide high-quality dental care to children, including those with special needs. Dr. Virdi has been running a specialized children's dental practice in Delhi since 2000. His practice is well known for its child-friendly environment and the use of the latest dental technology. Dr. Virdi has expertise in managing small children who require dental treatment under general anesthesia. He is a sought-after pediatric dentist in Delhi and the surrounding areas. Dr. Virdi is also associated with the Indian Dental Association (IDA). As an active member, he participates in various dental outreach programs and workshops to promote dental health and awareness among children and their parents. Dr. Virdi is also a professor and head of the Department of Pediatric Dentistry, PDM Dental College, Bahadurgarh, Haryana, India. He is known for his exceptional teaching skills and his commitment to providing his students with hands-on training and practical experience. Lastly, Dr. Virdi is actively involved in research. He has authored numerous research papers and articles in national and international dental journals. His research focuses on various aspects of pediatric dentistry, including dental trauma, behavior management, and dental caries.

Contents

Preface

Pediatric dentistry is a crucial aspect of dentistry that deals with oral healthcare for children, ranging from infancy to adolescence. The discipline encompasses the diagnosis, prevention, and treatment of oral diseases, as well as the promotion of oral health and well-being in children. The importance of pediatric dentistry cannot be overstated, as it ensures that children maintain good oral hygiene habits from a young age, which sets them up for a lifetime of good oral health.

This book provides a comprehensive overview of pediatric dentistry, focusing on several key areas. Chapter 1 discusses the concept of the "dental home," which refers to the ongoing relationship between a dentist and a child, beginning no later than the age of one. This concept ensures that children receive continuous, comprehensive oral healthcare that is tailored to their individual needs. Unfortunately, the dental home concept is often neglected in pediatric dentistry, resulting in poor oral health outcomes in children. This chapter highlights the importance of the dental home concept and its role in improving pediatric oral health.

Chapter 2 delves into the development of oral function in children, specifically focusing on a clinical study of stomatognathic dysfunction. Stomatognathic dysfunction refers to a range of disorders that affect the function of the oral cavity, including the teeth, jaws, and muscles. The chapter highlights the importance of early diagnosis and intervention in treating stomatognathic dysfunction in children, which can have long-term implications for their oral health and overall well-being.

Chapter 3 takes a community perspective on pediatric oral health, discussing the role of community prevention in promoting good oral health in children. The chapter provides an overview of community-based interventions, such as school-based oral health programs and community water fluoridation, and their impact on pediatric oral health outcomes. The chapter emphasizes the need for a collaborative approach to oral health promotion, involving dental professionals, community stakeholders, and policymakers.

Chapter 4 focuses on the effects of malnutrition on pediatric oral health. Malnutrition can have significant consequences on a child's oral health, including delayed tooth eruption, dental caries, and poor periodontal health. The chapter discusses the link between malnutrition and poor oral health outcomes in children, emphasizing the importance of proper nutrition in maintaining good oral health.

Finally, Chapter 5 examines the role of metals in pediatric oral health, specifically focusing on the use of metal-based restorative materials in pediatric dentistry. The chapter provides an overview of the different types of metal restorations, their advantages and disadvantages, and their impact on pediatric oral health outcomes. The chapter also discusses the use of metal-based orthodontic appliances in children and their potential impact on oral health.

In writing this book, I have relied on a range of sources, including peer-reviewed journal articles, textbooks, and clinical guidelines. I have taken care to ensure that all sources are properly cited and that the content presented in the book is accurate and current. I hope that this book will serve as a useful resource for dental professionals, students, and researchers interested in pediatric dentistry.

Mandeep Singh Virdi
Professor,
PDM Dental College and Research Institute,
Bahadurgarh, Haryana, India

Section 1

Preventive Pediatric Dentistry

Chapter 1

Perspective Chapter: Dental Home – A Neglected Primary Oral Health Care Concept

Krishna Patil, Rucha Davalbhakta, Buneet Kaur, Sujatha P, Smita Patil, Siddharth Shinde and Chetana Jagtap

Abstract

Tooth decay, if left untreated even in the earliest stages of life, can have serious implications for a child's long-term health and well-being. Early preventive care is a sound health and economic investment. Dental assessments and evaluations for children during their first year of life have been recommended by the American Academy of Pediatric Dentistry (AAPD) and the American Association of Pediatrics (ADA). Establishment of dental home and use of anticipatory guidance is one of the concepts in comprehensive oral health care. AAPD and ADA support the concept of a "dental home," which is the ongoing relationship between the dentist and the patient. Establishing a dental home means that a child's oral health care is managed in a comprehensive, continuously accessible, coordinated, and family-centered way by a licensed dentist. The dental professional's ability to provide optimal oral health care, beginning from when the child is 1-year-old, dental visit leading to preventive care and treatment as part of an overall oral health care foundation for life, is enhanced by dental home. The establishment of the dental home also assures appropriate referral to dental specialists when availability of direct care is not possible within the dental home.

Keywords: dental home, caries, neglected, primary health care, comprehensive

1. Introduction

The dental home for kids is the brand new idea for most of the dental career; however the concept of figuring out of child with the practitioner is acquainted for the scientific career. It provides evaluation to preventive and emergency services to kids.

Although oral health of kids residing in evolved international locations has been advanced drastically over beyond a long time still there are numerous youngsters in growing nations who preserve to suffer from oral sicknesses including caries, gingival infection and malocclusion. Early identification and management of the contributing factor play a crucial function now not handiest in prevention of oral ailment but additionally contributes for development of top of the line health within the children.

A only a few infants more youthful than 12 months have oral issues and require intervention, but almost all have an oral environment with the hazard of disease.

Early life caries have greater effects than caries taking place in person life as because of caries there is reduction in best frame weight of the child. It also represents sizeable economic and social burden and the timelines of preventive and early intervention is crucial for effective control (**Figures 1** and **2**).

Benefits of dental domestic have extended emphasis on prevention and ailment control, higher fitness effects at lower fee. Certain environmental factors may also impact the implementation of dental domestic [1].

"The dental domestic is the continuing dating among the dentist and the patient, which include all factors of oral health care brought in a complete, continuously handy, coordinated, and circle of relatives-centered way. Establishment of a dental home starts off evolved no later than twelve months of age and includes referral to dental professionals whilst appropriate" [2].

The dental home will offer a key message to the parents in addition to the care givers and it will likely be a notable for them to understand it and enforce it at the home level in preference to going to the dentist.

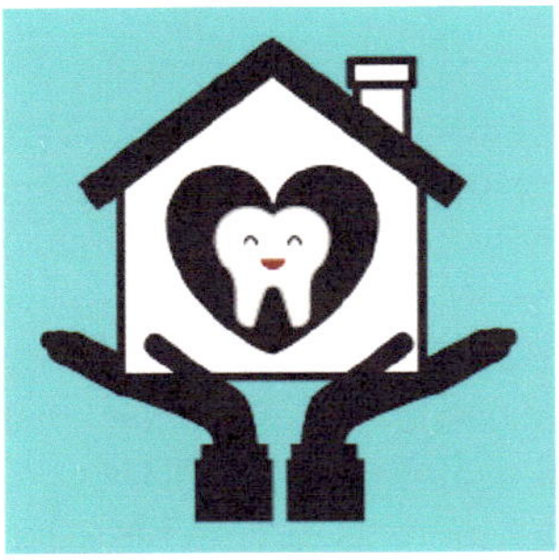

Figure 1.
Dental home.

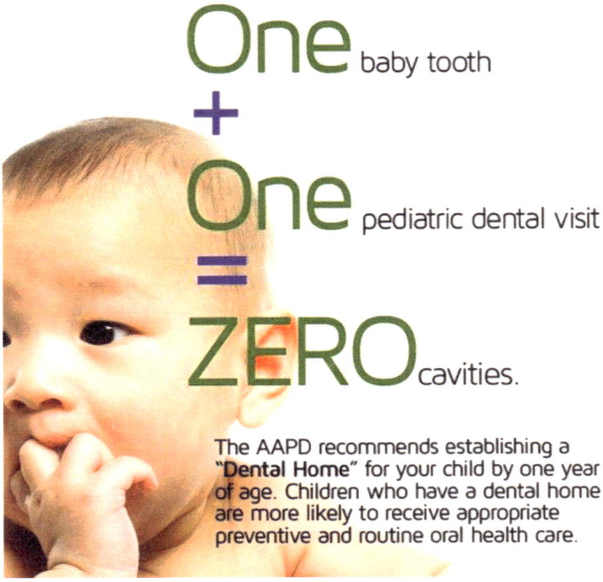

Figure 2.
Zero cavities.

2. Principles that guide the concept of dental home

2.1 The age one visit

The kid's first visit to the dentist should be when the first tooth erupts in the oral cavity preferably when first enamel erupts. When the child visits at the recommended age, a dental home can be set up and Anticipatory Guidance be established as a part of the kid's total health care [3].

In 1997 Nowak said that the first dental visit gives us information about the threat of dental sicknesses, it also offers anticipatory steering and decides the periodicity of future visits [4].

Predictive control, used in pediatric medicine, is a method of presenting realistic and developmentally relevant health data about a child to mothers and fathers in anticipation of important physical, emotional, and psychological milestones. Proactive guidance publications provide mothers and fathers with warnings about their next options, their role in maximizing their developmental potential, and their unique needs. The fact that it makes it recognizable. In the field of pediatrics, these active counseling criteria were introduced through well-child care visits. The information provided through predictive guidance is well understood by parents, as the process of interviewing by a pediatrician gives parents the opportunity to talk about their children and clarify their questions [5].

2.2 Anticipatory guidance in dentistry

This is a new paradigm for improving boom and development, caries prevention, and normal oral health. Preventive management in dentistry provides oral hygiene education, expert assessment, preventive measures, and nutritional advice from approximately 6 months to 2 years of age. This is step-by-step software that dentists are taught to those who actually seek care and are customized for each individual child. This is a time-consuming process consisting of oral testing, prevention, analysis of dietary plans, home care instructions, fluoride supplementation [both topical and systemic], and general feeding instructions [6].

Benefits of active consultation in dentistry:

a. Busy dentists and affected people will benefit from the positive control of the application.

b. The unique nature of this scientific software can be easily discovered by a scientific group of collaborators at all levels.

c. Predictive leadership establishes the interaction between the clinician and the parent.

d. Proactive Guidance solves the old-fashioned motivational problems encountered in traditional disease-based programs. Repeat the same simple message.

e. Active management of dental preventive education is for all dental companies to experience the eyes of dads and moms and to be more successful in preventive dentistry [7].

3. Need for dental home

- The emergence of social medication in pediatric health.
- Increasing knowledge about pediatric oral fitness danger and disease management.
- Dentistry as an independent career.
- Dental ability gadget for all kids together with youngsters with special dental care wishes.
- Perceived needs to dental care offerings and different boundaries that propels need for dental domestic utilization [8].

4. Mission of dental home

- An oral sickness unfastened populace.
- Availability of appropriate oral care for all children and sufferers with special health care desires.
- To be targeted on dental home [9].

5. Objectives

- To beautify dentists potential to teach sufferers and dad and mom or caregivers approximately the oral health.
- To schedule appointments for preventive strategies and explain the importance in phrases of oral fitness and value effectiveness.
- Evaluating hazard for dental sicknesses.
- Observing boom and improvement of the child.
- To give an explanation for the Importance of dental visits to the affected person and the parent.
- To refer patient to dental specialists for unique dental techniques [10].

6. Challenges in establishing a dental home

- Some dentists are hesitant to see youngsters under the age of six.
- Finding a dentist who is willing to work with families is difficult to come by.

- Covering the cost of dental services.
- Identifying resources for children who are uninsured.
- The price of care.
- Getting around transit and other roadblocks.
- Organizing transportation.
- Appointments that were not kept.
- Some remote areas have limited services.
- Persuading dad and mom to understand the importance of good oral hygiene [11].
- Younger children are cared for by dental professionals.
- A lack of understanding of current dental care.
- Negative personal gratification.

7. Services provided

A dental home must offer following offerings:

- Comprehensive oral care and acute care and prevention services.
- Comprehensive assessment of oral disorders and conditions.
- A personalized preventive dental care program based entirely on the caries risk assessment and the periodontal disease assessment.
- Positive guidance on the increase and development of problems (teeth, fingers, pacifier habits, etc.).
- Planning for acute tooth trauma.
- Information on proper care of children's teeth and gums. These may include prevention, analysis, and modification of destruction to supporting and surrounding tissues, as well as restoration of compatibility, function, and esthetics of these structures and tissues.
- Nutrition counseling.
- Referrals to dental specialists during dental treatment cannot be provided immediately.
- Education on future referrals to dentists [12].

8. Importance of dental home

It is gratifying to realize that we have the assist of the dental and health care community in our ongoing efforts to make sure first-rate oral health care of all our children. By organizing a dental home and taking preventive steps advocated by way of the pediatric dentist, mother and father can avoid their youngsters contracting early childhood caries—that is great devastating enamel decay that results in pain, failure to thrive, and in many instances, good sized and steeply-priced restorative work [13].

9. Some key findings

According to an article in Pediatrics, the authoritative magazine of the American Academy of Pediatrics, visiting children for oral health screenings and preventive services earlier saves money. The study looked at a cohort of 9200 Medicaid children in North Carolina between 1992 and 1997, and was spearheaded by Dr. Jessica Y. Lee of UNC-Chapel Hill. The average cost of a dental appointment for a child under the age of one is $262. This increased to $546, and the child's first visit was no longer till he or she was 4 years old. (These prices are based on the baby's spending over the course of the study, not on annual expenses) [14].

Medicaid-enrolled kids who had an early preventive dental visit had been much more likely to use next preventive offerings and revel in lower dental costs [15].

10. Characteristics of dental home

The following traits and there benefits so that it will be helpful for the uplifting of the dental domestic [16].

10.1 Accessible

Due to smooth of get right of entry to the care provided is in baby's network and it will likely be useful in coverage normal and adjustments in coverage accommodated.

The benefits can be that the source of care is near home and reachable to family. Minimal trouble encountered with price. Office is ready for treatment in emergency state of affairs. Office is nonbiased in coping with youngsters with unique health care needs. Dentist is aware of network desires and management.

10.2 Family focused

Recognition of centeredness of the circle of relatives is vital which enables to collect Unbiased complete records are shared on an ongoing bias.

This will help in low discern/child anxiety enhance care. Care protocols are secure to circle of relatives and suitable function of dad and mom in domestic care established.

10.3 Continuous

Same number one care is being supplied from infancy to formative years. Assistance furnished with transitions.

This will help in suitable bear in mind durations based on toddler's want.

Continuity of care is higher attributable to remember system versus episodic care.

Co-ordination of complicated dental remedy is possible.

10.4 Comprehensive

Health care will available 24 h consistent with day. Preventive, number one, tertiary care supplied. Emergency get entry to be ensured.

The Care supervisor and primary care dentist are in identical vicinity.

10.5 Co-ordinate

Families related to support, education and network services. Information and file is centralized.

School, workshop, remedy linkages are properly installed and known to all the members.

10.6 Compassionate

Expressed and confirmed difficulty for baby and family.

Dentist-toddler dating is set up.

Family relationship is mounted.

Children much less stressful thanks to familiarity.

10.7 Culturally competent

Cultural heritage diagnosed, valued, reputable.

Mechanism is mounted for communiqué for ongoing care.

Specialized sources are recognized and demonstrated if wished.

Staff can also talk other languages and realize dental terminology.

11. Steps taken when a patient approaches dental clinic

- History taking
- Detailed history taking allows achieving accurate prognosis.
- Clinical examination
- Thorough examination along with the intraoral and extra oral exam needs to be accomplished.
- Caries risk evaluation
- It is described as method to be expecting future caries improvement earlier than the clinical onset of the illnesses.
- Caries evaluation elements are

- Caries interest, demineralized regions, circle of relatives history, presence of plaque, fluoride exposure, sugar consumption, dental domestic, and many others.
- Caries evaluation Tools are Cariogram, traffic light matrix [17].

12. Advantages of dental home

- Access to dental home is close to the patient.
- Ready for treatment in emergency situation.
- Dentist knows community needs and resources.
- Co-ordination of complex dental treatment is possible.
- Embraces the importance of early intervention with optimal preventive strategies chosen based on the risk of the patient.
- Practitioner can provide personalized preventive approach for children.
- Dental home is to provide anticipatory guidance to the parents so that they are aware of children's growth and development [18].

13. Dental home in Indian scenario

In India, about 50% of children under the age of 5 and 80% of middle-aged people suffer from tooth decay. The incidence of dental diseases is high in India.

The fact that dentistry focuses on treatment rather than prevention. Expanding the scope of dental treatment (dentists, further training institutions) and technological advances have had little effect on actual prevention. Dental diseases are very preventable. However, it is widely believed that prevention is the responsibility of the government and its affiliates and is no longer a clinician practice. Definitive preventive techniques involving the addition of water fluoridation and the ban/replacement of sugar substances are no longer used in India due to the complexity associated with such issues. Therefore, the average person is often unaware of dental treatment and conveys ignorance (and sometimes frustration) about their oral problems that require complex treatment. The AAPD concept of dental homes can be called Indian dental homes. This is none other than a preventive dental clinic established to detect and prevent dental disorders that stand up in the circle of individuals or patients, and for loved ones. Preventive strategies in a special way [19].

We have a duty to provide people with sufficient and timely information on the prevention of dental diseases.

For example, a Preventive Dentistry Clinic must achieve the following goals:

a. Dental care should begin at a young age, with a focus on primordial and primary prevention.

b. Improving dentistry's reputation as a responsible profession.

c. The concept of health promotion.

d. Bridging the gap between the dentist and the general public in terms of communication.

The identification and removal of risk factors connected with a disease is considered primordial prevention.

14. Creation of awareness about prevention of oral diseases using concept of dental home

In order to render such preventive care, it's far important to satisfy parents/prospective parents early. Gynecologists, pediatricians, own family physicians are the folks who are available touch with them lots earlier than we do. We need to set up conversation with them such that powerful and timely referrals are made to preventive dentistry clinics.

Also, colleges and pre-school day care centers may be informed about the dental domestic idea or a preventive dentistry medical institution. A be aware consisting of—Do you know you may benefit your child's tooth and oral health with the aid of starting preventive dental care before baby-birth?—can attract the eye of prospective mother and father if installed a gynecologist's workplace.

We need to make preventative dentistry more accessible to the general public in a simple and effective way; for example,

A. A healthy smile for your baby can be achieved through preventive dentistry.

B. Children with healthy mouths can chew more easily and get more nutrients from the foods they eat.

C. They study how to speak extremely quickly and clearly.

D. They have a better possibility of achieving preferred fitness because a mouth sickness can jeopardize the body's relaxation.

E. A healthy mouth is more appealing, giving children self-assurance in their look.

F. Preventive dentistry entails a smaller and less expensive dental treatment for your child [20].

15. Key messages for the parent

1. First go to by the first birthday. Which will help in? Early exam and preventive care will shield your infant's smile now and within the future.

2. Tooth problems can start early. A major problem is early childhood cavities (also known as enamel cavities in baby bottles or breastfeeding cavities). Children can experience serious exacerbations when using bottles during naps, at night, or at some point after continuous breastfeeding.

3. The sooner you see your dentist, the higher your risk of preventing dental problems. Children with healthy tooth chew food easily, are higher capable of learn to talk in reality, and smile with confidence. Start kids now on an entire life of top dental behavior.

4. Encourage kids to drink from a cup as they technique their first birthday. Children ought to now not doze off with a bottle. At will nighttime breastfeeding have to be avoided after the first primary teeth start to erupt? Drinking juice from a bottle ought to be averted. When juice is obtainable, it should be in a cup.

5. Children need to be weaned from the bottle at 1214 months of age.

6. Thumb sucking is perfectly normal for babies; most stop by using age 2 and it ought to be discouraged after age 4. Prolonged thumb sucking can create crowded, crooked enamel or chunk issues. Dentists can advocate ways to deal with an extended thumb sucking dependency.

7. Do not soak in honey or sweets before giving the pacifier to your baby.

8. Limit the frequency of snacks. This may increase the risk of tooth decay in the baby.

9. Parents should ensure that the infant is of the right length, has a small cleaning surface, and uses a toothbrush that most effectively uses pea-sized fluoride toothpaste for each brushing. Toddlers should be monitored whenever they brush their teeth and taught to exhale rather than swallow toothpaste. Parents should not use fluoride toothpaste for children under the age of 2 unless recommended by a dentist or other fitness professional.

10. Children who generally drink bottled water may not be getting the fluoride they need.

11. From 6 months to 3 years of age, children may also suffer from periodontitis when they lose their teeth. Many children like smooth toothpaste, cold spoons, or bloodless wet washcloths. Some moms and dads choose chilled rings. Others rub the child's gums in good faith with clean fingers.

12. Parents and caregivers need to take care of their teeth so that the microbes that cause tooth decay are less likely to be transmitted to children. Do not clean with your own mouth before giving the pacifier or tableware to the child. It can also transmit bacteria from adults to children [21].

16. Conclusion

Dental domestic is an important idea for dentists to understand. The advantages of obtaining early career dental care and intervention are supported by evidence, which is supplemented by anticipatory advice for parents and frequent supervision visits based entirely on the child's risk of dental disorder. The dentist office should expand the availability of preventative oral health care for children in order to eliminate health disparities. The dental domestic concept, which warrants more examination and collaboration with the clinical domestic, would provide comprehensive health care to all children.

Author details

Krishna Patil[1*], Rucha Davalbhakta[1], Buneet Kaur[3], Sujatha P[2], Smita Patil[1], Siddharth Shinde[4] and Chetana Jagtap[1]

1 Department of Pedodontics, Bharati Vidyapeeth (Deemed to be University), Dental College and Hospital, Pune, Maharashtra, India

2 Department of Pedodontics, Bharati Vidyapeeth (Deemed to be University), Dental College and Hospital, Sangli, Maharashtra, India

3 Pedodontics, New Delhi, India

4 Department of Orthodontics, Bharati Vidyapeeth (Deemed to be University), Dental College and Hospital, Pune, Maharashtra, India

*Address all correspondence to: krishnapatil1000@gmail.com

References

[1] Nowak AJ, Casamassimo PS. The dental home A primary care oral health concept. Journal of the American Dental Association. 2002;**133**. DOI: 10.14219/jada.archive.2002.0027

[2] American Academy of Pediatric Dentistry. Available from: https://www.aapd.org/research/oral-health-policies\recommendations/Dental-Home/. [Accessed: October 19, 2021]

[3] Oral Health Risk Assessment Timing and Establishment of the Dental Home. American academy of pediatrics policy statement, organizational principles to guide and define the child health care system and/or improve the health of all children. Pediatrics. 2003;**111**(5). DOI: 10.1542/peds.111.5.1113

[4] Crall J, Silverman J. AAPD-OHS dental home initiative, overview partnering to provide dental homes and optimal oral health for HS/EHS children throughout the U.S. MSDA Symposium. 2009

[5] Nowak AJ. Pediatric Dentistry: Infancy Through Adolescence. 3rd ed. Philadelphia: Saunders; 1999. pp. 187-188. DOI: 10.1548/845214545.ch7

[6] Giriraju A. Nagesh Lakshminarayan dental home: A concept for early and everlasting smile: Review article. Scholars Journal of Dental Sciences. 2017;**4**(3):121-124. DOI: 10.21276/sjds.2017.4.3.8

[7] American Academy of Pediatric Dentistry. Policy on the Dental Home. The Reference Manual of Pediatric Dentistry. Chicago, Ill: American Academy of Pediatric Dentistry; 2020. pp. 43-44. Available from: https://www.aapd.org/media/Policies_Guidelines/P_DentalHome.pdf. [Accessed: October 19, 2021]

[8] McDonald and Avery's Dentistry for the Child and Adolescent. 7th ed. Chapter 11/247. DOI: 10.1588/514878955.ch7

[9] Hunke PH. The dental home and age one visit: The centerpiece of children's oral health care improvement. In: Presented to the Oral Health and School Readiness National Symposium. Vol. 18. 2016. Available from: https://issuu.com/peterjordan8/docs/dentalhome

[10] The Dental Home It's Never Too Early to Start American Dental Association. 2007. Available from: https://www.aapd.org/assets/1/7/DentalHomeNeverTooEarly.pdf. [Accessed: October 19, 2021]

[11] Building better oral health: A dental home for all Texans. A report commissioned by the Texas Dental Association. Tex Dental Journal Winter. 2008;(Suppl):1-56

[12] Thompson CL, McCann AL, Schneiderman ED. Does the texas first dental home program improve parental oral care knowledge and practices? Pediatric Dentistry. 2017;**39**(2):124-129. DOI: 39.22516/Peddent.2017.2.3

[13] Kolstad C, Zavras A, Yoon R. Cost-benefit analysis of the age one dental visit for the privately insured. Pediatric Dentistry. 2015;**37**(4):376-380. DOI: 376.2258/Peddent.2015.4.37

[14] Savage MF, Lee JY, Kotch JB, Vann WF. Early preventive dental visits: Effect on subsequent utilization and costs. Pediatrics. 2004;**114**:418-442. DOI: 10.1542/peds.2003-0469-F

[15] Grembowski D, Milgrom PM. Increasing access to dental care for Medicaid preschool children: The access to baby and child dentistry (ABCD) program. Public Health Reports. 2000;**115**:448-459. DOI: 10.1452/s0115-1452(4)445-9

[16] Tandon S. Text book of Pedodontics. 2nd ed. New Delhi: Paras Medical Publications; 2009. p. 227. DOI: 11.1252/5245896523.ch21. Chapter no 21

[17] American Academy of Pediatrics. Preamble to Patient Centred Medical Home Joint Principles. 2007. Available from: https://www.acponline.org/acp_policy/policies/joint_principles_pcmh_2007.pdf. [Accessed: October 20, 2021]

[18] Edelstein BL. Environmental factors in implementing the dental home for all young children. In: National Oral Health Policy Centre at Children's Dental Health Project. pp. 1-18

[19] Girish Babu KL, Doddamani GM. Dental home: Patient centered dentistry. Journal of International Society of Preventive and Community Dentistry. 2012;**2**(1):8-12. DOI: 10.4103/2231-0762.103448

[20] Ramos-Gomez FJ, Crystal YO, Ng MW, Crall JJ, Featherstone JDB. Pediatric dental care: Prevention and management protocols based on caries risk assessment. Journal of the California Dental Association. 2010;**38**(10):761. DOI: 11.1526/523322(10)746-61

[21] Nikhil M. Textbook of Pediatric Dentistry. 3rd ed. pp. 17-21. DOI: 11.1255/5245846523.ch3. Chapter 3

Section 2

Pediatric Dentistry

Chapter 2

The Development of Oral Functions in Children: A Clinical Study of Stomatognathic Dysfunction

Ichiro Nakajima, Ryosuke Koshi, Atsushi Uchida and Taketo Yamaguchi

Abstract

In most countries that have reached an aging society, the feeding function among the elderly population has declined and become a serious problem. Therefore, understanding the development of human oral function is required to address this problem. However, only a few research studies have reported oral motor functions and dysfunctions in children. Our chapter describes the relationship between oral motor functions (chewing, swallowing, and breathing) and maxillofacial morphology in children. In addition, case studies on children with cerebral palsy and sleep aspiration disorders will also be introduced. This study would also like to clarify the significance of human oral function development from infancy in pediatric dentistry.

Keywords: child, oral function, obstructive sleep apnea, cerebral palsy, achondroplasia

1. Introduction

Oral diseases include dental caries, periodontal (gum) disease, tooth loss, oral cancer, orodental trauma, and normal and birth defects such as cleft lip and palate [1]. These diseases have been known to be preventable by oral care [2]. Recently, most countries with aging societies implemented dental care significantly and strategically preventing age-related decline in oral functions [3, 4].

Oral health is a fundamental component of overall health. All children and youth should have access to preventive and treatment-based dental care. However, some children have difficulty availing of oral care and dental treatment due to their systemic disease or disability [5, 6]. Thus, caring and supporting for their oral functions remain unclear. Particularly, only a few studies have been conducted on the causes of oral dysfunctions in children with developmental motor dysfunction (i.e., cerebral palsy [CP], muscular dystrophy, etc.) and congenital malformation (achondroplasia, ectodermal dysplasia, etc.).

To clarify the relationship between systemic symptoms and oral dysfunction, symptoms of sensory-motor dysfunctions in CP and congenital malformation in achondroplasia have been examined, respectively.

Therefore, this chapter reviews the findings of previous studies and discusses the importance of establishing clinical research on oral dysfunctions in children with congenital diseases.

The contents of this chapter are as follows:

- Development of eating behavior
- Sensory-motor dysfunctions in the patients with cerebral palsy
- Obstructive sleep apnea in the children with achondroplasia

This chapter is believed to include useful content as a reference for clinical research on oral functions in children with disabilities.

2. Development of eating behavior

In this section, we briefly review the eating behavior development from the neonatal period in humans.

Oral functions consist of eating (breastfeeding and mastication), swallowing, and pronunciation/speech. The key to eating function development is the transition from breastfeeding to mastication behavior. Breastfeeding is an eating function composed of primitive reflexes, whereas mastication is a learning behavior composed of voluntary movement and chewing rhythm. In this section, we briefly describe the feeding function changes from the fetal to the neonatal to the weaning period.

2.1 Breastfeeding/suckle

The human jawbone is already formed around the 6th week of embryonic development. Moreover, the tooth germ formation of the primary teeth also begins around the 7th week. The calcification of the primary teeth begins around the 4th month. Since birth, a primitive reflex enables a newborn to suckle [7].

A newborn's oral cavity is sensitive and reflexive. For example, the sucking reflex is easily elicited by stimulating (tactile/chemical) the palate with the nipple.

- Rooting reflex: The reflex to seek the nipple
- Captive reflex: The reflex to catch the nipple
- Sucking reflex: The reflex to suck the mother's nipple with a fixed rhythm

The intermaxillary space and the presence of a sucking fossa in the palate are suitable forms for breastfeeding. During sucking, the tongue presses the nipple against the sucking fossa at the center of the palate (**Figure 1A**). The intermaxillary space is found in the anterior alveolar ridge of the upper and lower jaws before the primary tooth eruption. A newborn baby can use that space to hold the nipple (**Figure 1B**).

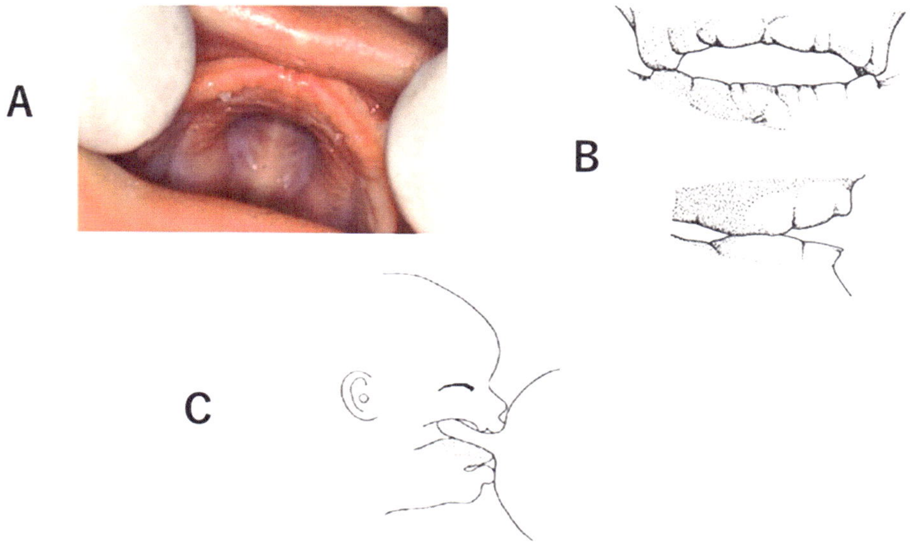

Figure 1.
Features of oral morphology for breastfeeding in newborns. A: sucking fossa, B: intermaxillary space, C: Tongue movement during breastfeeding.

The baby makes peristaltic movements from the tip of the tongue to the base of the tongue, creating negative pressure in the oral cavity and ingesting milk (**Figure 1C**).

Recently, Shiv Shankar Agarwal et al.'s cross-sectional retrospective study reported that children breastfed for <6 months had an almost twofold increased probability of developing sucking habits and non-spaced dentition than those who breastfed for >6 months duration [8]. Their data suggest the possibility that nonnutritive sucking habits may act as a dominant variable in the relationship between breastfeeding duration and occurrence of convex facial profile and disocclusion in deciduous dentition.

Furthermore, the study also evaluated the effects of breastfeeding and bottle feeding methods, such as bottle and cup feeding, on infant masticatory muscle activity, indicating that masticatory muscle activity is relatively high during breastfeeding. In any case, the oral function development in humans is thought to involve the suckling condition.

2.2 Mastication/chewing

Transitioning from sucking to mastication is a characteristic eating behavior change in mammals including humans. Tooth eruption and the associated stimulation from the surrounding tissue of the periodontal membrane are believed to be associated with the initiation of mastication (**Figure 2**). The weaning period is very important for the beginning of mastication.

At 5–6 months post-birth (weaning period), the upper and lower anterior teeth erupt, making it easier to separate the lip and tongue movements.

The changes observed during this period are as follows:

1. Expansion volume of the oral cavity.

2. Easier up and down movement of the tongue.

3. Mature swallowing with closing lips.

4. Crushing food with the tongue and alveolar ridge.

5. Crushing food with the teeth.

The upper and lower second primary molars erupt around age 2 years and 6 months, and the occlusion of 20 primary teeth is completed around 3 years (**Figure 3**).

With the second primary molar eruption, the masticatory force is believed to be increased. Biting force is further increased when the first permanent molars are occluded at 6 years, resulting in the establishment of mastication corresponding to growth during school age.

Recently, Nabeel et al. conducted a systematic review of jaw movements, bite force, and electromyograms of mastication from children aged <6–18 years [9].

They demonstrated that after 12 years, a significant increase in bite forces and electromyogram (EMG) activities occurred, and the frontal jaw pattern became similar to that of adults, suggesting that mastication gradually improves with the development of orofacial structures and was mainly influenced by a dental eruption.

As described in this section, an oral or stomatognathic function can be considered to be closely associated with nervous and muscular development as well as maxillofacial, oral cavity, and tooth growth.

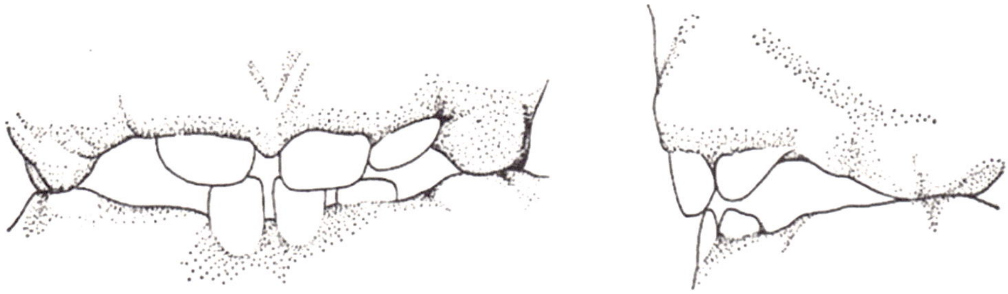

Figure 2.
Eruption of primary incisors.

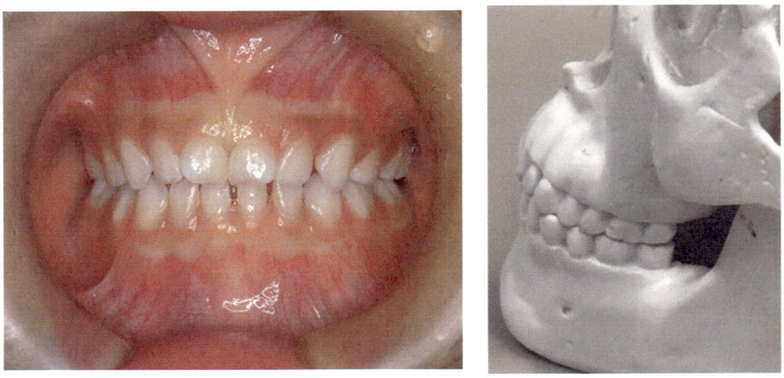

Figure 3.
Primary dentition occlusion.

3. Cerebral palsy (CP)

CP is a nonprogressive disorder that affects the motor system that moves the body due to a defect in the central nervous system (CNS). The defect might be before or at the time of or after the time of child's delivery [10]. The manifestation of CP is varied and depends upon the subtypes of CP. Motor system is the predominantly affected system with altered muscle tone, abnormal monosynaptic and polysynaptic reflexes, altered motor control and motor learning. The defects don't limit itself to the limbs and the trunk but also affect the face muscles, jaw muscles, which are closely associated with the head and neck muscles. Patients with CP were known to have lower feeding function than healthy subjects [11]. All clinical studies in this section were performed with ethics committee approval.

3.1 Masticatory efficiency and bite force

Nakajima et al. examined the relationships between masticatory efficiency, bite force, and masticatory rhythm in children with CP, comparing them with those in healthy children [12].

Table 1 shows the results of the comparison of masticatory efficiency and maximum bite force between children with CP and healthy children. The age ranges of children with CP and healthy children were 6–15 (mean age, 10) years) and 6–15 (mean age, 10) years, respectively. Adenosine triphosphate granules were used as mastication samples, and the amount of pulverization was measured based on absorbance.

	Masticatory efficiency	**Maximum biting force**
Children with Cerebral Palsy	0.167 ± 0.135	32.2 ± 20.8
Normal Children	0.545 ± 0.355	51.1 ± 16.0
Significant difference	**	**

Adapted from reference [12].

Table 1.
Comparison between children with cerebral palsy and healthy children in masticatory efficiency and maximum biting force.

As shown in **Table 1**, children with CP have significantly lower masticatory efficiency and bite force than healthy children of the same age. In the healthy children group, a significant correlation was also obtained with a correlation coefficient of 0.568 between the two indices ($p < 0.01$). Conversely, in children with CP, no significant correlation was observed with a correlation coefficient of −0.173 ($p > 0.05$).

These findings indicated that the muscle strength of mastication in CP may not be sufficiently developed to crush the mastication sample, as compared with their healthy counterpart.

Electromyogram (EMG) of the masticatory muscles (temporal and masseter muscles) during the masticatory efficiency measurement was recorded in the experiment. EMG data showed that children with CP had an unstable chewing rhythm compared to healthy children, suggesting an oral-facial sensation dysfunction that controls mastication.

3.2 Orofacial sensation

Patients with CP tend to develop accentuated involuntary muscle tonus in orofacial muscles during mastication. The muscle tonus abnormality is considered to affect oral sensation and a factor in reducing the eating function of patients with CP.

Therefore, Yoshida et al. investigated abnormalities in the lower-jaw-position sensation in patients using a lower-jaw-position discrimination test [13].

In that study, the mandibular position sensation was measured for adults with CP (CP group) and healthy adults (control group) using the following method.

This test was performed based on the extent of mouth opening to estimate a sensation associated with elongation of muscle spindles in masticatory muscles.

In the test, the participants were asked to hold a 10.0-mm metal rod (reference mouth opening) between the upper and lower incisors for several seconds and memorize its thickness. Thereafter, they were asked to hold another 0.5-mm-thick or thin metal rod and to answer whether these rods were "larger" or "smaller" than the standard mouth opening to count the wrong answers to examine the rate of miss estimate (RME).

Figure 4 shows the comparison between both groups based on RME data.

The RMEs of patients with CP were higher than those of healthy participants for jaw opening magnitudes, suggesting that some abnormalities exist in the mandibular sensation afferent system from the peripheral to CNS in patients with CP.

This phenomenon might be explained by the excessive excitation of the gamma motor nerves of muscle spindles, considering that the RME is extremely high at rods lower than the reference rod.

In other words, it is conceivable that patients with CP remain more sensitive to oral sensation than healthy participants.

Morimoto et al. reported that vibrating stimuli in healthy adults decreased the mandibular position sensation and considered that this phenomenon was caused by the regulation of the mandibular position sensation by muscle spindles [14]. Therefore, we also investigated the RME of mandibular position sensation by applying vibration stimulation to determine whether muscle sensory abnormalities in patients with CP are related to muscle spindles.

Figure 5 shows the comparison between both groups based on RME data after the vibration stimulation. No significant differences were observed between two groups for any interincisal distances ($p > 0.05$).

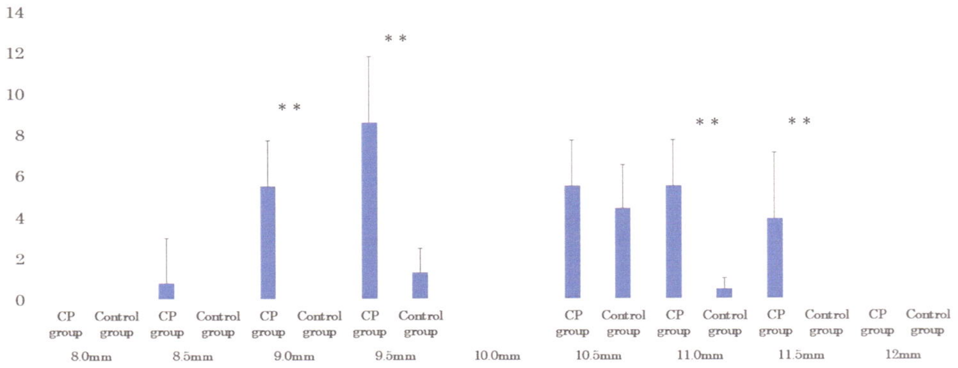

Figure 4.
Comparison between CP and control groups in R.M.E. for jaw position sense. Adapted from reference [13].

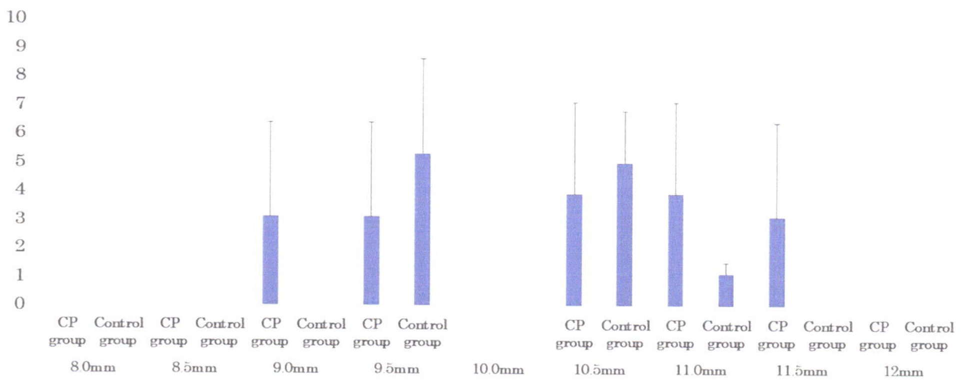

Figure 5.
Comparison between CP and Control groups in R.M.E of jaw position sense after vibration stimulation Adapted from reference [13].

When the discrimination ability of patients with CP was compared before and after the stimulus application, it was found to be significantly higher after the stimulation than before the stimulation when the interincisal distance was smaller (9.5 mm) than that with the reference stick ($p < 0.05$).

Conversely, in healthy participants, it was significantly lower after the stimulus than before the stimulus when the interincisal distance was smaller (9.5 mm) than that with the reference stick ($p < 0.05$).

Generally, it is known that following the application of vibration stimulus to voluntary muscles including the masticatory muscle and these muscles exhibit tonic vibration reflex (TVR) in which the muscles slowly shrink [14].

Vibration stimulation increases the excitability of muscle spindles and increases the impulse of GIa afferent nerve fibers. As the next step, monosynaptically connected alpha motor neurons are excited, causing continuous muscle contraction.

Assuming that TVR was expressed in both CP and control groups in the experiment, the result may suggest that the effect of TVR-induced muscle sensation was different between the two groups.

It was noteworthy that the discrimination ability in patients with CP increased by the vibration stimulation. Recently, vibration therapy is increasingly used to reduce signs and symptoms associated with this developmental disability [15]. These findings may support the effectiveness of these vibration therapies for orofacial muscles to improve oral functions in patients with CP.

3.3 Dental treatment and oral health care

Oral care and dental treatment are very important for patients with CP to maintain oral function. In dental clinics, patients with CP tend to accentuate involuntary muscle tonus in orofacial and other muscles when they must hold their jaw open, such as during teeth cleaning and dental treatment.

This abnormal muscle activity causes muscle fatigue and mental stress for patients.

Clinically, drug-induced sedation is used for patients with CP; however, no studies have examined its effects in detail. Therefore, to investigate how to control the muscle tonus, the authors investigated the effects of laughing gas (N2O) inhalation sedation on orofacial muscle tonus using EMG as an index [16]. In this study, the mean frequency of orofacial muscle EMG discharge was measured with other sedative indexes,

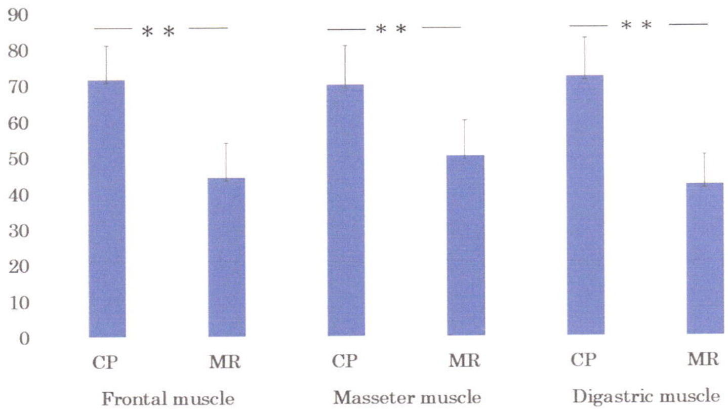

Figure 6.
The comparison of reduction rate of mean frequency between CP and MR groups during inhalation of N2O Adapted from reference [14].

blood pressure, and heart rate. The study patients were 15 patients with CP and 15 with mental retardation (MR) as the control. By forcing the jaw opening for dental treatment, the enhanced level of the mean EMG frequency was higher in patients with CP than in those with MR. After N2O inhalation, the mean frequency was significantly reduced in both patients with CP and MR.

Figure 6 shows the comparison of the reduction rate of mean frequency in patients with CP and MR. As shown in **Figure 7**, N2O selectively suppressed the muscle tonus in patients with CP.

In general, γ motor neuron blocking with phenol is a commonly used method to suppress accentuation of the limb skeletal muscles in patients with CP.

Therefore, hyperactivities of γ motor neurons may be involved in the increased muscle tonus of the orofacial area in patients with CP. The presence of muscle spindles has also been confirmed in the masseter muscle. However, the present study demonstrated that N2O also suppressed the muscle tonus in the frontalis and digastric muscles, which are thought to have no muscle spindles innervated by γ motor neurons.

Therefore, these results indicated the possibility that N2O suppressed the functions of the upper central nervous system related to the accentuation of the muscle tonus.

4. Obstructive sleep apnea in achondroplasia children

Sleep-related breathing disorders (SRBDs) during childhood are known to cause growth failure because of disturbed sleep and growth hormone secretion rhythm [18].

Furthermore, sleep-disordered breathing has also been found to affect brain development [18].

There is strong evidence that childhood SRBDs are associated with behavioral and emotional regulation, scholastic performance, sustained attention, selective attention, and alertness deficits. Failing to treat SDB appears to leave children at risk for long-term neurobehavioral deficits. Thus, a research platform has been created to validate the diagnosis and treatment of sleep apnea during childhood.

Obstructive sleep apnea (OSA) is classified as one of the SRBDs occurring when there are recurrent episodes of upper airway collapse and obstruction during sleep associated with arousals with or without oxygen desaturations.

Achondroplasia (hereinafter referred to as AP) is an autosomal dominant genetic disease with an incidence rate of 1 per 10,000 people.

There are abnormalities such as growth failure [19]. OSA symptoms have been reported in children with AP [20]. However, the relationship between OSA symptoms and maxillofacial morphology in children with AP is not yet sufficiently clarified. Therefore, A fact-finding survey on OSA symptoms for achondroplasia was implemented [21], and factors of maxillofacial morphology that cause apnea were analyzed using cephalometric X-ray data [22].

4.1 Respiratory symptoms and oral findings

A questionnaire survey was performed on a total of 30 children with AP (AP group), comprising 20 preschool and 10 school-aged children. The control group consisted of healthy kindergarten, primary school, and junior high school children to compare the incidence of snoring, apnea, mouth breathing, and malocclusion. Data from the control group were also obtained from the results of a questionnaire survey of kindergarten, primary school, and junior high school children, a survey of physical growth of preschool children, and a survey by the Japanese Society of Pediatric Dentistry. Except for the height and weight at birth, children aged 1.5 and 3 years were significantly smaller than those in the control group, except for the birth weight in the AP group.

Table 2 shows the incidences of snoring, apnea, mouth breathing, and cross/open bite at both preschool and school ages in the AP and control groups, respectively.

Group	Symptoms	Groups	Incidences	Significant difference
Preschool	Snore	Achondroplasia	95	**
		Control	5.9	
	Apnea	Achondroplasia	45	**
		Control	1.9	
	Mouth breathing	Achondroplasia	85	**
		Control	0.5	
	Cross-open	Achondroplasia	65	**
		Control	9.1	
School	Snore	Achondroplasia	90	**
		Control	60.6	
	Apnea	Achondroplasia	20	**
		Control	2.7	
	Mouth breathing	Achondroplasia	90	**
		Control	27.4	
		Control	27.4	
	Cross-open	Achondroplasia	60	**
		Control	9.2	

Adapted from reference [22].

Table 2.
Symptoms in children with achondroplasia.

At preschool age, the incidences of snoring, apnea, mouth breathing, and cross/open bite were significantly higher in the AP group than those in the control group, respectively ($P < 0.01$). At school age, the incidences of mouth breathing and cross/open bite in the AP group were significantly higher than those in the control group, respectively ($P < 0.01$). The incidence of snoring and apnea was higher than those in the control group, respectively ($P < 0.05$).

As a result of comparing the two groups, the AP group showed significantly higher incidences of snoring, apnea, mouth breathing, and reverse or open bite in infants and schoolchildren than those in the control group.

4.2 Craniofacial morphology (CFM)/airway morphology (AWM) in children with AP and healthy children

Figure 7 shows the measurement points of cephalometric photography.

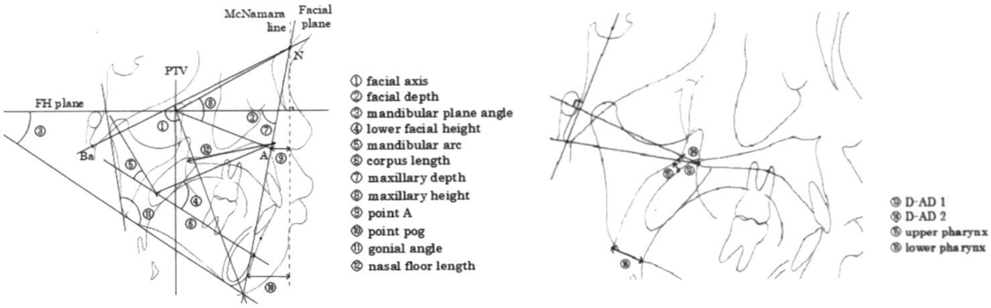

(A) (B)

Figure 7.
Measurement items (A) Maxillofacial morphology (B) Airway morphology. Adapted from reference [17].

Table 3 shows the comparison between children with AP and healthy groups in the measurement items of craniofacial/airway morphology.

In CFM, values for facial depth, nasal floor length, point A, point pog, and saddle angle were significantly lesser ($p < 0.01$), and those for mandibular plane angle and gonial angle were remarkably greater ($p < 0.01$) among AP group compared to the healthy. In AWM, D-AD1, D-AD2, and upper pharynx values were significantly lesser ($p < 0.05$among AP group.

These findings have been reported as common features in the unique facial features of children and adults with OSA [23].

The AP group showed CFM/AWM that was characteristic of upper airway stenosis, a retruded chin position, and a greater mandibular plane angle because of partial early ossification of the cranial bones and an greater lower facial height because of a greater mandibular angle. This suggests that that AP group will frequently encounter sleep snoring and sleep apnea compared to the healthy.

4.3 Diagnosis and treatment

In general, pediatric patients with achondroplasia undergo surgical procedures such as adenoidectomy and tonsillectomy in the field of otorhinolaryngology.

			Achondroplasia		Healthy		*p*-value
			Mean	S.D.	Mean	S.D.	
Craniofacial morphology	Significantly lower measurements	Facial depth	80.7	3.95	84.77	13.72	**
		Nasal floor length	43.03	3.37	48.2	1.97	
		Point A	−4.67	3.7	0.84	2.37	
		Point pog	−16.84	6.79	−8.62	3.31	
		Saddle angle	104.97	32.88	127.93	3.77	
	Significantly higher measurements	Mandibular plane angle	36.13	4.1	27.78	5.28	
		Gonial angle	135.61	6.8	126.27	7.45	
Airway morphology	Significantly lower measurements	D-AD1	8.3	3.43	17.08	4.34	**
		D-AD2	6.6	3.02	11.1	2.88	
		Upper pharynx	2.09	1.27	5.83	1.95	

Adapted from reference [17].

Table 3.
Morphological features of children with achondroplasia.

Sato et al. reported one case that adenoidectomy and tonsillectomy dilated the pharynx and improved the craniofacial and pharyngeal morphologies, apparently thus improving the sleep apnea [24].

A new diagnosis and treatment system for sleep apnea patients will be expected under the collaboration between pediatric dentistry and otolaryngology.

5. Conclusions

Clinical studies on developmental motor dysfunction are still limited. Further research developments that enable statistical review are warranted.

Acknowledgements

This work has received funding from the Nihon University School of Dentistry.

Conflict of interest

The authors declare no conflict of interest.

Notes/thanks/other declarations

We thank the staff of Nihon University Dental Hospital for their support.

Author details

Ichiro Nakajima[1*], Ryosuke Koshi[1], Atsushi Uchida[2] and Taketo Yamaguchi[3]

1 Department of Community Dentistry, Nihon University School of Dentistry, Tokyo, Japan

2 Department of Dentistry, Saitama, Japan

3 Department of Dentistry, Saitama Prefecture Kaikoen, Saitama, Japan

*Address all correspondence to: nakajima.ichirou@nihon-u.ac.jp

References

[1] WHO Publications. Oral health. [Internet]. 2022. Available from: https://www.who.int/health-topics/oral-health#tab=tab_1. [Accessed 2022-9-16]

[2] Peres MA, Macpherson LMD, Weyant RJ, Daly B, Venturelli R, Mathur MR, et al. Oral diseases: A global public health challenge. Lancet. 2019;**394**(10194):249-260. DOI: 10.1016/S0140-6736(19)31146-8

[3] Patel J, Wallace J, Doshi M, Gadanya M, Yahya IB, Roseman J, et al. Oral health for healthy ageing. Lancet. 2021;**2**(8):e521-e527. DOI: 10.1016/S2666-7568(21)00142-2

[4] Zaitsu T, Saito T, Kawaguchi Y. The oral healthcare system in Japan. Healthcare. 2018;**6**(3):79. DOI: 10.3390/healthcare6030079

[5] Ningrum V, Bakar A, Shieh TM, Shih YH. The oral health inequities between special needs children and normal children in Asia: A systematic review and meta-analysis. Healthcare (Basel). 2021;**9**(4):410. DOI: 10.3390/healthcare9040410

[6] Obeidat R, Noureldin A, Bitouni A, Abdellatif H, Miranda SL, Liu S, et al. Oral health needs of U.S. children with developmental disorders: A population-based study. BMC Public Health. 2022;**22**:e861. DOI: 10.1186/s12889-022-13237-2

[7] Watanabe S. Development of masticatory function. Dental, Oral and Craniofacial Research. 2017;**3**(7):1-2. DOI: 10.15761/DOCR.1000S2004

[8] Agarwal SS, Nehra K, Sharma M, Jayan B, Poonia A, Bhattal H. Association between breastfeeding duration, non-nutritive sucking habits and dental arch dimensions in deciduous dentition: A cross-sectional study. Progress in Orthodontics. 2014;**15**(1):59. DOI: 10.1186/s40510-014-0059-4

[9] Almotairy N, Kumar A, Trulsson M, Grigoriadis A. Development of the jaw sensorimotor control and chewing - A systematic review. Physiology and Behavior. 2018;**194**:456-465. DOI: 10.1016/j.physbeh.2018.06.03

[10] Bobath K. A Neurophysiological Basis for the Treatment of Cerebral Palsy. London: William Heinemann Medical Book; 1980

[11] Weir KA, Bell KL, Caristo F, Ware RS, Davies PS, Fahey M, et al. Reported eating ability of young children with cerebral palsy: Is there an association with gross motor function? Archives of Physical Medicine and Rehabilitation. 2013;**94**(3):495-502. DOI: 10.1016/j.apmr.2012.10.007

[12] Nakajima I, Ohnishi T, Nagasawa A, Seki M, Takanashi N, Takei K, et al. Relationship between the values of masticatory efficiency and biting pressure in children with cerebral palsy. The Journal of Nihon University School of Dentistry. 1980;**30**(3):244-260. DOI: 10.2334/josnusd1959.30.244

[13] Yoshida M, Nakajima I, Uchida A, Yamaguchi T, Nonaka T, Yoshida H, et al. Characteristics of lower-jaw-position sensation with respect to oral-jaw functions in patients with cerebral palsy. Pediatric Dental Journal. 2004;**14**(1):23-28. DOI: 10.11411/pdj.14.23

[14] Morimoto T, Kawamura Y. Conditioning-effect of vibratory stimulation on dimension discrimination

of objects held between human tooth arches. Archives of Oral Biology. 1976;**21**(3):219-220. DOI: 10.1016/0003-9969(76)90133-3

[15] Ritzmann R, Stark C, Krause A. Vibration therapy in patients with cerebral palsy: A systematic review. 2018;**14**:1607-1625. DOI: 10.2147/NDT.S152543

[16] Yoshida M, Nakajima I, Uchida A, Yamaguchi T, Akasaka M. Effect of nitrous oxide on dental patients with cerebral palsy -- Using an electromyogram (EMG) from orofacial muscles as an index. Journal of Oral Rehabilitation. 2003;**30**(3):324-333. DOI: 10.1046/j.1365-2842.2003.00979.x

[17] Chiba S, Ashikawa T, Moriwaki H, Tokunaga M, Miyazaki H, Moriyama H. The influence of sleep breathing disorder on growth hormone secretion in children with tonsil hypertrophy. Nihon Jibiinkoka Gakkai Kaiho. 1998;**101**(7):873-878. DOI: 10.3950/jibiinkoka.101.7_873 abstract in English

[18] Isaiah A, Ernst T, Cloak CC, Clark DB, Chang L. Associations between frontal lobe structure, parent-reported obstructive sleep disordered breathing and childhood behavior in the ABCD dataset. Nature Communications. 2021;**12**:2205. DOI: 10.1038/s41467-021-22534-0

[19] Pauli RM. Achondroplasia: A comprehensive clinical review. Orphanet Journal of Rare Diseases. 2019;**14**:1. DOI: 10.1186/s13023-018-0972-6

[20] Sisk EA, Heatley DG, Borowski BJ, Leverson GE, Pauli RM. Obstructive sleep apnea in children with achondroplasia: Surgical and anesthetic considerations. Otolaryngology–Head and Neck Surgery. 1999;**120**(2):248-254. DOI: 10.1016/S0194-5998(99)70414-6

[21] Onodera K, Sakata H, Niikuni N, Nonaka T, Kobayashi K, Nakajima I. Survey of the present status of sleep-disordered breathing in children with achondroplasia Part I. A questionnaire survey. International Journal of Pediatric Otorhinolaryngology. 2005;**69**(4):457-461. DOI: 10.1016/j.ijporl.2004.11.005

[22] Onodera K, Niikuni N, Chigono T, Nakajima I, Sakata H, Motizuki H. Sleep disordered breathing in children with achondroplasia. Part 2. Relationship with craniofacial and airway morphology. International Journal of Pediatric Otorhinolaryngology. 2006;**70**(3):453-461. DOI: 10.1016/j.ijporl.2005.07.016

[23] Tanimoto Y, Miyamoto K, Sugiyama A, Tanne K. Incidence of snore and association with craniofacial morphology in growing patients with malocclusions. The Journal of Hiroshima University Dental Society. 2000;**32**:94-101. Available from: https://ir.lib.hiroshima-u.ac.jp/00016951. (in Japanese)

[24] Sato K, Niikuni N, Nakajima I, Shirakawa T, Sakata H. Surgical treatment for sleep apnea: Changes in craniofacial and pharyngeal airway morphology in a child with achondroplasia (case report). Journal of Oral Science. 2007;**49**(2):173-177. DOI: 10.2334/josnusd.49.173

Chapter 3

Perspective Chapter: Oral Health and Community Prevention in Children

Irma Fabiola Díaz-García, Dinorah Munira Hernández-Santos, Ana Bertha Olmedo-Sánchez and Luz Elena Nápoles-Salas

Abstract

The child population is the most affected by the presence of caries. A preventable disease, which causes pain and school absenteeism, generates a significant expense in its treatment. If left untreated, it causes early tooth loss and malocclusion. Altering the quality of life at an early age leaves sequels. Primary care is essential in the prevention of oral diseases. Contact with the health team in first-level medical units, which begins during pregnancy and continues in the following stages of the child, plays an important role in its prevention, diagnosis, and treatment. Across the health system, these primary care practitioners play an important role in children oral health which includes provide preventive care, referral to dentists or dental care providers and caries risk assessment. This team will know how to refer the child to the dentist specialized in the treatment. This strategy largely represents community prevention. To this must be added the family, and the school, making use of the promotion of oral health in favor of children. Efforts to prevent childhood dental caries cannot only focus on individuals and their biology and behaviors individually. It should consider the backup determinants of children's dental health as well.

Keywords: oral health, community prevention, early childhood caries, primary care, preventive dental care

1. Introduction

Children have the right to health and to enjoy their childhood in the best possible way. Healthy children have better opportunities to grow, develop, and learn and later become healthy and productive adults [1].

Child health should be understood as the necessary capacity for children or groups of children to develop and reach their potential, satisfy their needs, and develop the talents that allow them to successfully interact with their biological, physical, and social environment [2].

The period of childhood covers between 0 and 18 years. The notion of health status is different during childhood than in adulthood. Due to their development, children have a constant dynamic in their health and are exposed during this time to multiple biological, environmental, cultural, and behavioral influences. It may be that these influences become risk or protective factors and/or promoters of health [1].

Oral health plays a primary role in the physical, mental, social, and economic well-being of individuals and populations. The oral cavity and the structures that surround it are essential parts of the human body, an integral part of its daily functioning, and contribute substantially to the general well-being of people [3]. All children and youth should have access to preventive services and treatment-based dental care [4].

Oral health promotion plays a fundamental role in the promotion of general health, since the interrelation between oral and general health has been approved [5]. Oral health promotion aimed at the entire child population is the general objective of a public dental health system. According to the United Nations Convention on the Rights of the Child, every child has the right to good oral health [6].

The presence of caries in children increases the risk of infections, malocclusion, and feeding and language difficulties, impacting school absenteeism, general health, and family finances [7]. In addition, the presence of untreated caries is another of the great problems faced by the child population. Statistical data show that in 2015, 7.8% of the global child population (573 million children) had untreated dental caries. The prevalence of untreated caries in deciduous and permanent teeth peaks at ages 1 to 4 years and 15 to 19 years, respectively [8]. Early childhood caries (ECC) remains the most common chronic childhood disease, with almost 1.8 billion new cases per year worldwide. It affects approximately 37% of children aged 2 to 5 years in the United States, and up to 73% of socioeconomically disadvantaged preschool children in both developing and industrialized countries [9].

2. Primary health care

Primary health care (PHC) is one of the most important measures to promote the health of the population, and it represents "essential medical care". The interventions are scientifically proven. It focuses on equitable distribution, community participation, an emphasis on prevention, the use of appropriate technology, and the involvement of a wide range of other health departments [10].

The concept of primary health care (PHC) was defined at the Alma Ata conference in 1978. After the conference, the concept of PHC was gradually developed during the 1980s by the health promotion approach. Health promotion according to the WHO (1984) includes the following points: 1) health promotion involves the population as a whole, in the context of their daily lives, rather than focusing on people at risk of specific diseases; 2) it is aimed at action on the determinants or causes of health; 3) combine diverse, but complementary, methods or approaches; 4) it aims at a particularly effective and concrete public participation; and 5) health professionals have an important role in fostering and promoting health [11].

2.1 Primary health care and oral health

The evolution of this paradigm caused that, in 2009, at the seventh world conference of the WHO, dental care was integrated into primary health care services. It includes several domains, such as risk assessment, oral health assessment, preventive intervention, communication and education, as well as interprofessional collaborative practice [12].

The integration of oral health into primary care has been implemented in some health care systems to reduce the burden of oral disease and improve the access to oral health care, especially for disadvantaged individuals and communities [13].

2.2 Primary care and oral health in children

In primary health care, interprofessional collaboration provided by medical personnel is a very helpful preventive strategy for children's oral health. Medical providers have numerous opportunities to see children from birth to at least 3 years old. On average, there will be 12 visits on a regular basis during this time; the medical office is a space that serves to extend access to preventive oral health services for children. Basic preventive oral care that may be provided by the physician includes as follows: 1. oral health risk assessment; 2. anticipatory oral health guidance; 3. application of fluoride varnish; 4. dental referral; and 5. prescription of fluoride supplements [12].

From the point of view of primary oral health care, what should be considered "essential" oral health care is crucial, especially in developing countries [11]. Children who had an early preventive dental visit were more likely to use preventive services later and incur lower dental costs over time [4].

The preventive services offered by the PHC are of great importance for oral health, and many mothers in the gestation stage are first attended by health workers in these centers, such as gynecologists, family doctors, nursing assistants (midwives), and activists accredited socio-sanitary, are people who come into contact with them long before a dentist. So, they can identify oral problems, such as the presence of tooth decay before a dentist. The dental surgeon must establish communication with them in such a way as to make an effective and timely referral to the dental outpatient department of a nearby public/private hospital. Therefore, it is important to meet expectant mothers/fathers-to-be at an early stage.

Untreated dental caries in mothers increases the risk of caries development among their children, as maternal transmission and early caries in children have been established. Vertical colonization of Streptococcus mutans from mother to child is well documented. Studies have shown that these Streptococcus are initially acquired by children from their mothers at around 2 years of age, which is the window of infectivity [14].

Primary care physicians frequently see children with pain due to dental cavities, as well as increased school absenteeism, eating problems, sleep loss, and risk of serious infections. The American Academy of Pediatrics (AAP) has recommended that primary care health care professionals conduct oral health risk assessments beginning at 6 months of age and refer patients to a dentist at 12 months of age [15].

2.3 Primary health care and children with special needs

For children with special care needs and for their parents, APS will help in the prevention and control of many oral ailments. Infants and children with special health care needs may be at increased risk of developing oral conditions such as delayed tooth eruption, malocclusion, tooth decay, dental abnormalities, trauma, infections, and enlarged gums. It is very important that a general health professional is aware of these conditions and makes a referral to the appropriate dental specialist.

All of the conditions these children experience are attributed to various congenital syndromes, medications, or inherent immune deficiencies and include Down syndrome, Treacher-Collin syndrome, and ectodermal dysplasia. Various medications cause gingival enlargements; for example, dilantin (phenytoin sodium) and phenobarbital, which are prescribed for epilepsy, can cause gingival hyperplasia. It is very important that a general health professional is aware of these conditions.

These children may need regular dental referrals. Like all children, they should have their first visit within 6 months after the eruption of the first tooth or at 12 months of age. However, future visits may need to be more frequent [14].

3. Community prevention

Oral Health Promotion Programs (OHPP) for children are implemented globally in various communities and have been shown to be a useful intervention to control dental caries [5]. Dentists and oral health providers prioritize oral health promotion through education and prevention programs for all family members, children and parents, at all socioeconomic levels. Since they are the only means to avoid dental caries [16].

Unfortunately, dental programs and oral health prevention programs rarely receive the same level of attention as medical care among decision-makers when cost-effective allocation of scarce health resources is taken into account. This occurs despite statistics showing a high prevalence of oral diseases.

The 2016 Global Burden of Disease Study estimated that oral diseases affect at least 3.58 billion people worldwide. Dental caries is the most prevalent chronic disease among children, and dental care is the largest uncovered health care need [5]. It is a major public health problem [4].

3.1 Working together for health

Community participation in disease prevention is part of primary health care. To understand what it consists of, it is essential to recognize that the health of individuals and groups is defined by multiple factors, some of these determinants are very close and others far from individual control, in addition to this, there are social inequalities in health, that is, a distribution unequal opportunity to enjoy health. The impact of interventions on the different levels of health determinants is variable. Thus, policies (macroeconomic, employment, rights, etc.) influence more and more people than interventions closer to individuals [17].

Evidence of the importance of social determinants makes health a collective issue. This statement has two implications. The first is that although medical services can improve health, this is not a consequence of medicine but of all its determinants, one of which, but not the only one or the most important, is health services. The second is that health services must be reoriented to incorporate the collective dimensions of health and to address modifiable determinants from their sphere of social responsibility [18].

Oral health does not escape social determinants, for example, the population in contexts of poverty, social exclusion or low educational level, is more frequently exposed to unhealthy hygienic-dietary habits, and this situation is observed in relation to the presence of dental caries due to its multifactorial nature. Certain dietary habits increase the risk of appearance, while the frequency of brushing decreases it in the permanent dentition [7].

In the child population, oral health disparities are well documented, with low-income minority children experiencing the highest prevalence and disease of caries [19]. In some low- and middle-income countries, the presence of caries in children aged 5 to 6 years exceeds 90%, indicating that dental caries is a permanent public health problem [5].

Evidence shows that childhood caries is associated with impaired cognitive development, increased school absenteeism, poorer school performance, increased job loss for parents, and poorer quality of life [19].

For this reason, simultaneous action at various levels is of the utmost importance, to enhance the effects of health interventions, so it is convenient to align the actions on the person and their immediate environment, such as the family and the place of study or work, with those that act further away from it, such as the policies that influence the neighborhood, the workplace, or the municipality.

Community work in favor of health is a network, and it consists of creating alliances to establish shared objectives and act cooperatively to achieve them. This network must include not only the different services involved (intersectionality) but also the community itself (community participation), since the commitment of each other will facilitate the implementation and maintenance of changes [17].

3.2 Preventive community strategies for oral health in children

Preventive dental care can significantly improve oral health in children [20]. Interventions that integrate the participation of health and non-health sectors have been shown to be more effective in preventing diseases, since they cover the complexity of the problem, promoting awareness, autonomy, and the involvement of family networks among groups of increased risk [7].

3.2.1 The school and the family main actors in community health

There is more evidence that schools and parents are needed to reinforce good practices in children. Good oral health practices in the first 5 years of a child's life are critical to lifelong oral health. Factors including toothbrushing, fluoridation, dietary advice, and visiting the dentist, among others, improve oral health and behavior [21].

Since childhood caries is a public health problem, the WHO emphasizes the urgent need to act to control it and suggests its population-based prevention, through educational interventions on oral health (such as avoiding free sugars in complementary foods and beverages, promoting breastfeeding, using toddler finger brushes or soft brushes for children twice a day) aimed at pregnant women, new mothers, and primary health care providers, as well as interprofessional education with other health professions.

The family plays an essential role in interventions to improve brushing in young children. A clear example is the result of research, which shows that toothbrushing behaviors of young children are strongly associated with those of their parents, or caregivers, and with the level of family support for brushing [19].

Various factors have been identified that affect dental caries in children, including poor oral hygiene and nutritional status, as well as the level of knowledge, habits, attitudes, and self-efficacy related to oral health among school teachers and parents. These variables must be taken into account when developing oral health education programs for preschool children.

Oral health education can be reinforced throughout the school years, an influential period in children's lives. Lifelong beliefs, positive attitudes, and personal skills develop among children during the school years. During the children's school career, oral health education should be promoted in all their courses. In addition, it must be regularly reinforced at home with school programs designed for it. School staff and parents should be involved in the school's oral health promotion efforts [22].

3.2.2 Dental and non-dental staff

In addition, it recommends that, in order to bring childhood caries prevention measures closer to a greater number of children, they should be planned at appropriate times, such as the vaccination period. There is also a need to develop a training package for dental and non-dental staff to provide adequate prevention and management of this disease. On the other hand, interventions aimed at mothers, both during pregnancy and in the first year after childbirth, can effectively prevent this condition in a critical way [23].

3.2.3 Use of fluorides

The combination of community, professional, and individual measures to control the caries process in children is the most effective strategy, for example, promoting proper nutrition, improving diet, fluoridating water, increasing the use of topical fluorides and dental sealants by primary health care providers, and using fluoride toothpaste.

The most effective public health preventive measure against caries is water fluoridation. The cost benefit is undeniable. The application of topical fluorides in the form of varnish in children reduces caries rates, proven by strong scientific evidence. Evidence recommends twice-yearly varnish application for high-risk populations, including indigenous children. Regular use of fluoride mouth rinses has been shown to reduce dental caries in older children, independent of other sources of fluoride [4].

4. Integration of oral health in general medical care: the pediatrician our ally

Oral health is an indicator of overall health, quality of life, and well-being. Most oral diseases and conditions share modifiable risk factors with major noncommunicable diseases, such as cardiovascular disease, cancer, chronic respiratory disease, high levels of stress, and diabetes. There is a proven relationship between oral and general health. It is reported, for example, that diabetes is related to the development and progression of periodontitis. In addition, there is a causal link between high sugar consumption and diabetes, obesity, and tooth decay [24].

Pediatricians are the custodians of children's overall health and are the ideal health care staff to impart information and instructions on oral health care to this child population. This is mostly due to the number of children seen by pediatricians, which is much higher than what general dentists see. However, it is a responsibility that must be shared between these three professions, the dentist, the pediatrician, and the general practitioner. Many of the aspects that pediatricians can observe and that may go unnoticed by dentists are issues such as diet, weight, maturation, vaccines, different diseases, and growth [25].

4.1 Gap in pediatric knowledge about oral health

Pediatricians have begun to play an important role in promoting oral health in their patients, taking preventive measures such as monitoring, referral to dental services, and prior oral health counseling. However, it must also be recognized that there is also some limitation on the part of pediatricians, both in knowledge and in understanding certain clinical areas that are critical. This include differentiating the first clinical signs of dental caries, which is the recommended age to go to the dentist for the first time, the transmission of bacteria from the mother to her baby as part of the etiology of caries, and the use of fluoride [26].

The problem is serious because, if pediatricians do not identify certain factors, they will not refer these patients to a dentist, which has the consequence that there is no preventive care, and this being an important element for the oral care of children. To this is also added that sometimes the communication between the pediatrician and the dentist is not completely coordinated. This is because many pediatricians do not consider referring patients to the dentist as a necessity as soon as oral ailments are detected [27].

5. Oral health disparities at an early age

Oral diseases in children are an urgent public health problem worldwide. It is estimated that early childhood caries affects around 600 million children worldwide, but this condition is entirely preventable. Dental health professionals around the world must act to improve the use of prevention measures and quality dental health care to improve global oral health [28].

Most children in the United States have benefits for having good oral health, such as a socially acceptable smile, frequent visits to the dentist directly, as well as not suffering from pain in their teeth. Many of them have the health insurance that parents have, which partially covers the cost of treatment [29].

In a systematic review in which 72 articles were included, it was determined that the prevalence of early childhood caries amounted to 98%, being present in children ranging from 4 to 12 years of age [30]. Mainly the groups of children with low socioeconomic status and people with a lower degree of education are affected. Oral diseases are expensive to treat, which is why they seriously affects the most disadvantaged population [31].

5.1 Social gradients in health

Different studies show a strong association between economic position and the prevalence of oral diseases, which has been named "social gradient in health" [32].

While social gradients in perceived oral health and overall health exist in adult and child populations, not many studies have evaluated whether social gradients exist in a low-income population, specifically in a community of low-income mothers and their young children. It is important to know this perspective from the course of life, since mothers are the main source of transmission of tooth decay bacteria to their children. If there are social gradients in the oral health of low-income mothers, these gradients can be passed on to their young children and persist into adulthood [33].

Policies should focus on improving oral health education, as this could lessen gradients in oral health in low-salary mothers and their kids. Strong connection has been found between maternal-dental education and general health. If associations are causal, attempts to rise the education of low-income mothers can lead to have a better progress in their oral health. This result can break with the pattern of transmission of health gradients from education to their young children [34].

Children who are in this economic situation experience longer dental appointments to repair or remove teeth that are in an unfavorable state; in turn, they are patients who experience pain or who may be dealing with a picture of infection. These patients are usually taken to dental care under emergency and not as prevention [29].

5.2 Disparities by race and ethnicity

An ethnic group is defined as a group of people who identify with each other based on their affinities, such as the language itself, ancestral, social, national, cultural experiences, gastronomy, and religion [35].

Taking into account internationalization and the increase in migrant groups, the number of children of non-native origin will grow even more in the future, and with it the possibility of an increase in inequalities in oral health [36].

It has been reported that race and ethnicity also represent an important stratification factor for oral health disparities, as a result of an unbalanced distribution of dental services and care, as well as the economic situation among different racial communities. These groups are severely affected by tooth loss, lack of oral hygiene, tooth decay, and eating difficulties, among others [37].

There is an important theoretical and empirical literature on ethnic inequalities in health, which considers how exclusionary social processes such as labor market segregation, unemployment, income inequality, and poverty disproportionately affect racialized and immigrant groups and translate into health disparities [38].

Another difference that has been found depending on the community to which you belong is when choosing dental treatment. For example, African Americans are less likely to choose endodontic treatment than Hispanics. Also due to their economic situation, degree of education, and access to dental health, they report having worse access to oral health, a very bad perception of oral health and a high prevalence of dental caries. Language also plays an important role in gaining access to dental health. Namely, in the United States, people who do not speak English very well can face different barriers, which brings repercussions for their health [39].

5.3 Actions to improve inequality in oral health

Currently, there is considerable evidence that inequalities in oral health are attenuated with the passage from childhood to adolescence. This socioeconomic stabilizaton in health during puberty is thought to improve when the impact of the family and family environment decrease, and that school, peers, and youth culture have a special role in children's lives [40].

Puberty is a phase when behaviors related to oral health are not supervised as closely by parents as they are during infancy. School and neighborhood potentially play a bigger role that can influence oral health and related behaviors. In addition, the transition from childhood to adolescence is a period of sensitive development in oral health, a stage that is accompanied by the replacement of primary teeth with permanent teeth. A reduction in tooth decay in early adolescence may mean less lifelong exposure of permanent teeth to oral health risk factors [41].

According to The Lancet, dentistry is in crisis globally: "Current dental care and public health responses have been largely inadequate, inequitable and costly, leaving billions of people without access to even basic public oral health care" [42].

Public policies and programs focused on children's oral health generally have two main objectives: to diminish the effect of oral conditions on the community and to lessen obstacles that restrict access to oral health services. Exemplifications are potable water, fluoridation, and education programs aimed to improve and promote oral health literacy and as a result a healthy behavior. It also includes surveillance actions to supervise trends and identify high-risk-need groups and programs that supply screening and preventive services in schools or other community spaces [43].

6. Risk factors for oral diseases at an early age

Oral health is a situation that affects both children and young people and the elderly. Efforts to improve oral health should be supported by research that includes socioeconomic, biological, and demographic factors, which increase susceptibility to develop oral diseases. Birth cohorts are longitudinal studies in which follow-up is performed from birth. This type of study is scarce, and in oral health much more. There are currently four different studies of this type: the one in the city of Pelotas in Brazil, the longitudinal study of Australian children, the Christchurch health and development study, and the Dunedin multidisciplinary development and health study [44].

The results of this study show us that various factors are involved for the development of dental caries in childhood, whether protective or risky. Oral health education and the use of dental services are influenced by the belief mainly of parents that it is not necessary to go to this type of assistance until the child starts school [44].

Tooth decay is a multifactorial disease that is affected by cariogenic plaque, fermented carbohydrates, time, a susceptible tooth, environmental factors such as saliva, fluoride availability, dental knowledge of parents, access to dental care, and socioeconomic issues [45].

The type of diet consumed in the child population plays a very important role. The intake of foods with high sugar content represents a great risk to oral health and consequently, for the subsequent development of oral diseases. These are easy to acquire, being able to generate among other aspects, caries, diabetes, hypertension, and obesity. The risk factors require a time of exposure to them to be able to cause some oral damage in individuals; that is why, at an early age, many damages cannot be easily observed, so you have a period where apparently there is no disease [46].

Malocclusions are one of the oral diseases that most affect the population, because they are multifactorial. The appearance of a malocclusion at an early age represents an indicator that this disease can be maintained at other ages and/or condition the appearance of others. This condition, in addition to causing morphofunctional damage, leaves the individual more susceptible to trauma. Several studies report that the presence of an increased highlight in children was a risk factor for suffering a traumatic injury [47].

7. Oral health from childhood and healthy aging

Oral health in childhood and early childhood play a very important role, as they are precursors of good oral health later in life. That is why children have been the main objective to promote oral health and to develop scopes to prevent oral diseases. Many resources have been researched for a better understanding of the factors that affect oral health in children, primarily preschool children, mothers, and caregivers (National Institute of Dental and Craniofacial Research [48].

As more studies show us about the effects of early-life experiences, experts are focusing on prevention and medical care, including activities that promote oral health during preconception, pregnancy, and the first 3 years of life. Health promotion activities represent a key element in decreasing morbidity, mortality, improving overall health and wellbeing [48].

A significant body of scientific evidence has established a strong relationship between oral health, overall health, and healthy aging. These tests are clear enough to justify their application in public health programs, in dental establishment, and in local groups in ways to promote healthy aging. The implementation of policies favorable to oral health would represent an effective and efficient use of public financial resources [49].

Aging is a serious global health problem for low-, middle-, and high-income countries. As we encourage the prolongation of life expectancy, this turns out as a monumental challenge. With age, a person becomes more vulnerable to the disease, and this leads to decreased intrinsic ability and functional ability [50].

It is not possible to achieve healthy aging without providing all people with access to the services and education that are necessary to maintain oral health and the functions we perform with it: eating, talking, and smiling. In ways to delay functional decline and rise people's health and well-being, it will be important not only to provide medical attention and long-term care insurance for all but also to include these systems of care into a much wider social infrastructure that therefore stimulate healthier behaviors [50].

8. Conclusions

Primary care plays a key role in the prevention of oral diseases in childhood. All primary care workers must direct their efforts so that children do not suffer from any oral disease or are diagnosed and treated early. On many occasions, they are the first contact with the future mother, with the new mother, and with the children in their early childhood. Therefore, their collaboration is invaluable to promote oral health in the family and in children.

Involve people, families, community leaders, health care practitioners, educators, and policy-makers will help in the making of a framework to be used in and with the community. Addressing disparities is recognized as a crucial part of improving oral health. This can be more efficient when used in a culturally sensitive framework that addresses concerns particular to specific communities.

Community prevention as part of primary health care involves the whole of society. The public and private health sector, the school, and the family are essential actors in health promotion. We all have the commitment to ensure a future with well-being for children. A child free of oral conditions is a child with a better chance of developing healthily.

Conflict of interest

"The authors declare no conflict of interest."

Author details

Irma Fabiola Díaz-García*, Dinorah Munira Hernández-Santos,
Ana Bertha Olmedo-Sánchez and Luz Elena Nápoles-Salas
Universidad de Guadalajara, Guadalajara, Jalisco, México

*Address all correspondence to: irma.dgarcia@academicos.udg.mx

References

[1] Pérez-Cuevas R, Muñoz-Hernández O. Importancia de la salud pública dirigida a la niñez y la adolescencia en México. Bol. Med. Hosp. Infant. Mex. 2014;**71**(2):126-133

[2] National Research Council (US). Institute of Medicine (US). Children's Health, the Nation's Wealth: Assessing and Improving Child Health. Washington (DC): National Academies Press (US); 2004. DOI: 10.17226/10886

[3] National Institutes of Health. Oral Health in America: Advances and Challenges. Bethesda, MD: US Department of Health and Human Services, National Institutes of Health, National Institute of Dental and Craniofacial Research; 2021

[4] Rowan-Legg A. Canadian paediatric society, community paediatrics committee. Oral health care for children - a call for action. Paediatrics & Child Health. 2013;**18**(1):37-50. DOI: 10.1093/pch/18.1.37

[5] Fraihat N, Madae'en S, Bencze Z, Herczeg A, Varga O. Clinical effectiveness and cost-effectiveness of Oral-health promotion in dental caries prevention among children: Systematic review and Meta-analysis. International Journal of Environmental Research and Public Health. 2019;**16**(15):2668. DOI: 10.3390/ijerph16152668

[6] Nydell Helkimo A, Rolander B, Koch G. Dental fear in school children and young adults attending public dental health care: Prevalence and relationship to gender, oral disease and dental treatment; trends over 40 years. BMC Oral Health. 2022;**22**(1):146. DOI: 10.1186/s12903-022-02166-6

[7] Calderón Larrañaga S, Expósito Ruiz M, Cruz Vela P, Cuadrado Conde A, Alquézar Villarroya L, Garach Gómez A, et al. Primary Care and oral health promotion: Assessment of an educational intervention in school children. Aten Primaria. 2019;**51**(7):416

[8] Kanagaratnam S, Schluter PJ. A review of dental caries in adolescents, risk factors and preventive strategies. New Zealand Dental Journal. 2021;**117**(1):5-13

[9] Xiao J, Alkhers N, Kopycka-Kedzierawski DT, Billings RJ, Wu TT, Castillo DA, et al. Prenatal oral health care and early childhood caries prevention: A systematic review and Meta-analysis. Caries Research. 2019;**53**(4):411-421. DOI: 10.1159/000495187

[10] Bourgeois DM, Phantumvanit P, Llodra JC, Horn V, Carlile M, Eiselé JL. Rationale for the prevention of oral diseases in primary health care: An international collaborative study in oral health education. International Dental Journal. 2014;**64**(Suppl. 2):1-11. DOI: 10.1111/idj.12126

[11] Honkala E. Primary oral health care. Medical Principles and Practice. 2014;**23**:17-23. DOI: 10.1159/000357916

[12] Prasad M, Manjunath C, Murthy AK, Sampath A, Jaiswal S, Mohapatra A. Integration of oral health into primary health care: A systematic review. Journal of Family Medicine Primary Care. 2019;**8**(6):1838-1845. DOI: 10.4103/jfmpc.jfmpc_286_19

[13] Harnagea H, Lamothe L, Couturier Y, Esfandiari S, Voyer R,

Charbonneau A, et al. From theoretical concepts to policies and applied programmes: The landscape of integration of oral health in primary care. BMC Oral Health. 2018;**18**(1):23. DOI: 10.1186/s12903-018-0484-8

[14] Suresh KS, Kumar P, Javanaiah N, Shantappa S, Srivastava P. Primary Oral Health Care in India: Vision or dream? International Journal of Clinical and Pediatric Dental. 2016;**9**(3):228-232. DOI: 10.5005/jp-journals-10005-1369

[15] Dooley D, Moultrie NM, Heckman B, Gansky SA, Potter MB, Walsh MM. Oral health prevention and toddler well-child care: Routine integration in a safety net system. Pediatrics. 2016;**137**(1):e20143532. DOI: 10.1542/peds.2014-3532

[16] Colombo S, Paglia L. Part 1: Prevention first. European Journal of Paediatric Dentistry. 2018;**19**(1):80-82. DOI: 10.23804/ejpd.2018.19.01.15

[17] Isabel PM, Elia D. Salud comunitaria: una actuación necesaria. Gac Sanit [Internet]. 2013;**27**(6):477-478. DOI: 10.1016/j.gaceta.2013.10.001

[18] Montaner I, Foz G, Pasarín MI. La salud: ¿un asunto individual? AMF. 2012;**8**:374-382

[19] Martin M, Pugach O, Avenetti D, Lee H, Salazar S, Rosales G, et al. Oral health Behaviors in very young children in low-income urban areas in Chicago, Illinois, 2018-2019. Preventing Chronic Disease. 2020;**17**:E152

[20] Hannan CJ, Ricks TL, Espinoza L, Weintraub JA. Addressing Oral health inequities, access to care, knowledge, and Behaviors. Preventing Chronic Disease. 2021;**25**(18):E27. DOI: 10.5888/pcd18.210060

[21] Henderson E, Rubin G. A model of roles and responsibilities in oral health promotion based on perspectives of a community-based initiative for pre-school children in the U.K. British Dental Journal. 2014;**216**(5):E11. DOI: 10.1038/sj.bdj.2014.196

[22] Shirzad M, Taghdisi MH, Dehdari T, Abolghasemi J. Oral health education program among pre-school children: An application of health-promoting schools approach. Health Promotion Perspective. 2016;**10**(3):164-170

[23] Deghatipour M, Ghorbani Z, Mokhlesi AH, Ghanbari S, Namdari M. Community-based interventions to reduce dental caries among 24-month old children: A pilot study of a field trial. BMC Oral Health. 2021;**21**(1):637. DOI: 10.1186/s12903-021-01999-x

[24] Organización Mundial de la Salud. Oral Health. 2022. Available https://www.who.int/health-topics/oral-health#tab=tab_1

[25] Goyal A, Nishant MR, Gauba K, Jaiswal M. Awareness among pediatricians regarding oral health care in children including those with special health care needs: A cross- sectional survey. Journal of Family Medicine and Primary Care. 2020;**9**:4151-4155. DOI: 10.4103/jfmpc.jfmpc_539_20

[26] Dickson-Swift V, Kenny A, Gussy M, et al. The knowledge and practice of pediatricians in children's oral health: A scoping review. BMC Oral Health. 2020;**20**:211. DOI: 10.1186/s12903-020-01198-0

[27] Quinonez RB, Kranz AM, Long M, Rozier RG. Care coordination among pediatricians and dentists: A cross-sectional study of opinions of North Carolina dentists. BMC Oral Health. 2014;**14**:33

[28] Ramos-Gomez F, Kinsler J, Askaryar H. Understanding oral health disparities in children as a global public health issue: How dental health professionals can make a difference. Journal of Public Health Policy. 2020;**41**(2):114-124. DOI: 10.1057/s41271-020-00222-5

[29] Crall JJ, Vujicic M. Children's Oral health: Progress, policy development, and priorities for continued improvement. Health Affiation. 2020;**39**(10):1762-1769. DOI: 10.1377/hlthaff.2020.00799

[30] Tinanoff N, Baez RJ, Diaz-Guillory C, et al. Early childhood caries epidemiology, aetiology, risk assessment, societal burden, management, education, and policy: Global perspective. International Journal of Pediatric Dental. 2019;**29**:238-248. DOI: 10.1111/ipd.12484

[31] Acuña-González GR, Casanova-Sarmiento JA, Islas-Granillo H, Márquez-Rodríguez S, Benítez-Valladares D, Mendoza-Rodríguez M, et al. Socioeconomic inequalities and toothbrushing frequency among schoolchildren aged 6 to 12 years in a multi-site study of Mexican cities: A cross-sectional study. Children (Basel). 2022;**18**(7):1069

[32] Peres MA, Macpherson L, Weyant RJ, Daly B, Venturelli R, Mathur MR, et al. Oral diseases: A global public health challenge. Lancet. 2019;**394**:249-260. DOI: 10.1016/S0140-6736(19)31146-8

[33] Poulton R, Caspi A, Milne BJ, Thomson WM, Taylor A, Sears MR, et al. Association between children's experience of socioeconomic disadvantage and adult health: A life-course study. Lancet. 2002;**360**:1640-1645. DOI: 10.1016/S0140-6736(02)11602-3

[34] Grembowski D, Spiekerman C, Milgrom P. Social gradients in dental health among low-income mothers and their young children. Journal of Health Care for the Poor and Underserved. 2012;**2**:570-588. DOI: 10.1353/hpu.2012.0054

[35] Isajiw WW. Definitions of ethnicity. Ethnicity. 1974;**1**(2):111-124

[36] Stoeldraijer L, van Duin C, Huisman C. Bevolkingsprognose 2017-2060: 18,4 miljoen inwoners in 2060. Technical Report December. Den Haag: C

[37] Bastos JL, Celeste RK, Paradies YC. Racial inequalities in Oral health. Journal of Dental Research. 2018;**97**(8):878-886. DOI: 10.1177/0022034518768536

[38] Shi C, Faris P, McNeil DA, Patterson S, Potestio ML, Thawer S, et al. Ethnic disparities in children's oral health: Findings from a population-based survey of grade 1 and 2 schoolchildren in Alberta, Canada. BMC Oral Health. 2018;**18**(1):1. DOI: 10.1186/s12903-017-0444-8

[39] Kelesidis N. A racial comparison of sociocultural factors and oral health perceptions. Journal of Dental Hygiene. 2014;**88**(3):173-182

[40] Rouxel P, Chandola T. Socioeconomic and ethnic inequalities in oral health among children and adolescents living in England, Wales and Northern Ireland. Community Dentistry and Oral Epidemiology. 2018;**46**(5):426-434. DOI: 10.1111/cdoe.12390

[41] Bernabe E, Delgado-Angulo EK, Murasko JE, Marcenes W. Family income and tooth decay in US children: Does the association change with age? Caries Research. 2012;**46**:221-227. DOI: 10.1159/000337389

[42] Lancet Press Office. The lancet: Big sugar and neglect by global health community fuel oral health crisis. The Internet. 2019. Available: https://www.eurek alert.org/pub_relea ses/2019-07/tl-tlb07 1619.php

[43] Crall JJ. Federal support for oral health care: The long view. Journal of Public Health Dentistry. 2012;**72**(1):S61-S62

[44] Hong CL, Broadbent JM, Thomson WM, Poulton R. The Dunedin multidisciplinary health and development study: Oral health findings and their implications. Journal of the Royal Society of New Zealand. 2020;**50**(1):35-46. DOI: 10.1080/03036758.2020.1716816

[45] Chen KJ, Gao SS, Duangthip D, Lo ECM, Chu CH. Early childhood caries and oral health care of Hong Kong preschool children. Clinical, Cosmetic and Investigational Dentistry. 2019;**11**:27-35. DOI: 10.2147/CCIDE.S190993

[46] Kirthiga M, Murugan M, Saikia A, Kirubakaran R. Risk factors for early childhood caries: A systematic review and Meta-analysis of case control and cohort studies. Pediatric Dentistry. 2019;**41**:95-112

[47] Torres S, Barberán D, Bruzon D, Figueredo E, Rosales G. Factores predisponentes de trauma dental en escolares del municipio Rafael Freyre. CCM. 2017

[48] National Institute of Dental and Craniofacial Research (US). Oral Health in America: Advances and Challenges. Bethesda (MD): National Institute of Dental and Craniofacial Research

[49] Fukai K, Dartevelle S, Jones J. Oral health for healthy ageing: A people-centred and function-focused approach. International Dental Journal. 2022;**72**(4S):S2-S4. DOI: 10.1016/j.identj.2022.06.001

[50] World Health Organization. World report on ageing and health. The Internet. 2015. Available: https://apps.who.int/iris/handle/10665/186463

Section 3

Nutrition and Oral Health

Chapter 4

Perspective Chapter: Effects of Malnutrition on Pediatric Oral Health – A Review

Kempaiah Siddaiah Madhusudhan and M.R. Pallavi

Abstract

Malnutrition occurs when there are deficiencies, excesses, or imbalances in a person's intake of energy and or nutrients. Diet and nutrition affect oral health in several ways. Early childhood malnutrition is in association with dental caries, enamel hypoplasia, salivary gland hypofunction, and delayed eruption. Poor oral health is in association with tooth decay, periodontal disease, and lesions in other oral tissues among children and older adults. This correlation between malnutrition adversely affects the oral structures and poor oral health, which in turn, leads to poor nutrition (Malnutrition). Various nutritional deficiencies, along with deficiencies of protein, energy foods, or both affect the development of the oral cavity. Dietary practices, nutritional status, general health status, and oral health conditions are all interrelated factors. Due to malnutrition, there are multiple effects on the oral tissues and subsequent development of oral disease. This paper gives an insight into the interrelationship of malnutrition affecting the development of the oral cavity and the progression of the oral disease.

Keywords: Malnutrition, Oral cavity, PEM (protein energy malnutrition), enamel hypoplasia, pediatric oral health

1. Introduction

Nutrition is the intake of food, considered in relation to the body's dietary requirement. Good nutrition is an appropriate, well-balanced diet combined with regular physical activity which is a keystone of good health. Poor nutrition (Malnutrition) can lead to reduced immunity, increased susceptibility to disease, impaired physical and mental development, and reduced productivity.

Malnutrition is the condition that develops when the body does not get the right amount of vitamins, minerals, and other nutrients that it needs to maintain healthy tissues and organ functions. Deficiencies of protein, energy foods or both which are relative to body's needs leads to Protein-Energy Malnutrition (PEM) [1, 2]. Malnutrition affects oral health and poor oral health, therefore, leads to malnutrition. Good nutritional health aids good oral health and vice versa, this interrelationship between good oral health and good nutritional health leads to homeostasis. Malnutrition alters this homeostasis leading to decrease resistance to the microbial

 IntechOpen

biofilm, decrease in immune response and capacity of tissue healing is lowered. Malnutrition leads to disease development in the oral cavity [3].

Studies have indicated that enamel hypoplasia, saliva compositional changes, and salivary gland hypofunction may be the mechanisms by which malnutrition is associated with caries, where altered eruption timing may create a challenge in the analysis of the age-specific caries rates [3]. Malnutrition is wide-ranging in rural, tribal, and urban slum areas. Malnourishment in children is due to adverse cultural practices, destruction of the environment, gender inequality, inaccessible medical care, lack of education, large family size, overpopulation and poverty [4]. Poor oral health, including tooth decay, periodontal disease and lesions in other oral tissues among older adults can profoundly diminish quality of life and have an adverse impact on general health [5, 6].

2. Oral cavity and its structural manifestations in nutritional status of the body

Nutrition is the study of how food affects the body. It is the adequate provision of materials like vitamins, minerals, fiber, and water and other food components to cells and organisms, to support life. Many common health problems can be prevented or alleviated with good nutrition [7].

"Malnutrition is the cellular imbalance between the supply of the nutrients and the energy and the body's demand for them to ensure growth, maintenance, and specific functions" [8].

The oral cavity is influenced by the diet for development, depending on whether there is an early or late nutritional imbalance, the consequences are certainly different. A shortage of minerals and vitamins in the conception period influences the development of the dental organogenesis in the future embryo, the growth of the maxilla, and skull/facial development. Early nutritional disproportion influence malformations at most. Diet influence the health of the oral cavity, conditioning the onset of caries, development of the enamel, the onset of dental erosion, state of periodontal health, salivary characteristics, and oral mucous in general [9].

There exist a strong interconnection between poor oral health and malnutrition. Poor oral health such as missing teeth or gum disease leads to inability in chewing or swallowing food can negatively impact nutritional intake (e.g., children tend to consume soft, fewer and lower nutritional value meals) leading to poor nutritional status and increased risk of malnutrition [10, 11]. Malnourished children lack proper nutrients leading to increased risk of oral health related disease which can negatively impact oral health related quality of life [3]. PEM (Protein Energy Malnutrition) is of mild, moderate and severe type. Such malnutrition status during development of the body can affect the oral structure also (**Table 1**) [1].

Nutritional status of the body influence the pre-eruptive phase of the teeth. The deficiencies of vitamin D, vitamin C, vitamin B, and vitamin A and Protein Energy Malnutrition (PEM) have been associated with disturbances in the oral structures. Enamel hypoplasia are the hypoplastic grooves and/or pits, which is often horizontal or linear in appearance which is a characteristic of the lesion [1]. Enamel hypoplasia and pits correlate to a lack of vitamin A. More diffused hypoplastic forms of the enamel have been reported with a vitamin D deficiency as well [12, 13]. The structural damage can testify to the period in which the lack of nutrition has occurred.

Nutritional deficiencies such as vitamin B and iron deficiencies causes the conditions like recurrent aphthous stomatitis, atrophic glossitis, or a painful, burning tongue

Deficient Nutrient	Effect on oral structures
Protein/calorie Malnutrition	Delayed tooth eruption, Reduced tooth size Decreased enamel solubility, Salivary gland dysfunction.
Vitamin A	Decreased epithelial tissue development, Impaired tooth formation, Enamel hypoplasia.
Vitamin D/Calcium Phosphorus	Lowered plasma calcium, Hypomineralization Compromised tooth integrity, Delayed eruption pattern Absence of lamina dura, Abnormal alveolar bone patterns.
Vitamin C	Irregular dentin formation, Dental pulpal alterations, Bleeding gums, Delayed wound healing, Defective collagen formation.
Vitamin B1(Thiamine)	Cracked lips, Angular cheilosis
Vitamin B2 (Riboflavin) Vitamin B3 (Niacin)	Inflammation of the tongue, Angular cheilosis, Ulcerative gingivitis
Vitamin B6	Periodontal disease, Anemia, Sore tongue, Burning sensation in the oral cavity.
Vitamin B12	Angular cheilosis, Halitosis, Bone loss, Hemorrhagic gingivitis, Detachment of periodontal fibers, Painful ulcers in the mouth
Iron	Salivary gland dysfunction, Very red, painful tongue with a burning sensation, Dysphagia, Angular cheilosis

Table 1.
Effects of malnutrition on the oral cavity and its structures.

which is characterized by inflammation and defoliation of the tongue [7, 10, 14]. In maintaining the healthy oral cavity, salivary gland function should be normal. In PEM it has been reported that there will be salivary gland hypofunction, which results in a decreased salivary flow rate, a decreased buffering capacity, and decreased salivary constituents, particularly proteins [1, 15]. PEM and vitamin A deficiency are associated with salivary gland atrophy which leads to reduce defense capacity against infection and buffering ability to plaque acids [15].

Host factors are also associated with the development of caries, delay in the exfoliation and the eruption [16], especially tooth defects and the salivary system in PEM. Malnutrition was not associated with crowding, but crowding was seen in permanent dentition only in mouth-breathing adolescents [17]. The tooth defects on external structural defects (hypoplasia) provide a more cariogenic environmental niche and less protective enamel, which might increase the susceptibility to demineralization. The salivary flow rates are related to caries directly through oral clearance and in terms of the buffering capacity and the antimicrobial components [1]. Periodontal disease evolves more quickly in undernourished populations. The most important risk factor in the development of periodontal disease is represented by inadequate oral hygiene. Malnutrition and bad oral hygiene represent the two important factors that predispose to necrotizing gingivitis [12].

3. Discussion

The onset of the malnutrition is early during the intrauterine life or childhood, or it can occur during an individual's lifetime as a result of poor nutrition [16]. Malnutrition is a multifactorial. Deficiencies of protein, vitamin D and vitamin A have been associated with enamel hypoplasia. Vitamin A deficiencies and protein energy malnutrition are commonly associated with salivary gland atrophy. Protective Role of saliva, its amount and composition, buffering capacity, defense against infection in oral cavity is reduced and manipulated during salivary gland atrophy [13].

Deficiency of B-complex vitamins also affects oral structures. Burning sensation in the mouth is a common oral effect of B (complex) deficiency, especially on the tongue. Inflammation of the lining of the oral cavity and the tongue, oral ulcers, cracks at the corners of the mouth (angular cheilitis), cracked and red lips, and a sore throat are the other oral symptoms of B-complex deficiencies. The effects of vitamin B deficiency and iron deficiency are similar. To produce healthy red blood cells within the bone marrow the body requires iron, vitamin B12, and folic acid. Deficiency of B-complex vitamins like B12 or folic acid results in pernicious anemia, a condition in which there will be increased number of immature red blood cells in circulation. Riboflavin (vitamin B2) is primarily required for the breakdown of the lipids, ketone bodies, carbohydrate, and proteins. However, ariboflavinosis manifests as cracked lips, dryness, glossitis, glossodynia and glossopyrosis due to vitamin B2 deficiency [7, 14, 18–20].

In a study, moderate to severe PEM had reduced salivary secretion rate, reduced buffering capacity, lower calcium levels, a lower protein secretion in stimulated saliva, and reduced agglutinating defense factors in unstimulated saliva was found in Indian children [21]. In a retrospective cohort study which was designed by Psoter et al. found a continued effect on the diminished salivary gland function into adolescence, which was a result of Early Childhood Malnutrition (EC-PEM). In EC-PEM, the exocrine glandular systems may be compromised in body's systemic antimicrobial defenses [15].

Two cross-sectional studies inferred that malnutrition in children not only cause a delay in tooth exfoliation and eruption but also renders the deciduous teeth more susceptible to a caries attack later in life [22, 23]. Another retrospective cohort study showed the evidence of tooth exfoliation/eruption patterns and a nutritional insufficiency (stunting) throughout childhood. There was a delayed exfoliation of the primary tooth and eruption of permanent [16].

Density of the alveolar bone that supports the teeth is determined by the calcium similar periodontal health by vitamin C. Connective tissue repair and its healthy maintenance along with antioxidant properties are the main role of vitamin C. Scurvy a clinical condition due to deficiency of vitamin C is characterized by defective collagen synthesis. Bleeding gums and gingivitis are the main oral manifestations of scurvy [7, 24, 25].

Older adults are at an increased risk of malnutrition and poor oral health. In a study, older patients were screened in three emergency departments (ED) for malnutrition and contributing risk factors, including oral health [26]. A separate study found that over 25% of older patients screened for malnutrition in a dental clinic were malnourished or at risk [27].

These reviews, further support malnutrition and oral health are interrelated. Importance should be given when considering health related problems in children, older adults in healthcare, dental care and social services.

4. Recommendations

1. Breastfeeding should be initiated within 1 hour of the delivery [28].

2. Exclusive breastfeeding importance for the first 6 months and proper weaning thereafter has to be explained to the mothers.

3. Importance of consumption of a cost effective nutritious diet has to be imparted to people through nutritional education.

4. Importance of the family planning and adequate spacing between children should be promoted for limiting the family size and to improve the standard of living.

5. Under nutrition can be halted by promoting proper environmental sanitation.

6. Tackling of malnutrition mainly depends on the rural socioeconomic development.

7. Improvement of the health sectors through integrated health packages should be initiated; in this regard government should allocate more funds.

Incorporate screening for malnutrition and oral health into practice to provide better care and support to children, older adult patients, and clients. It is evident from the present review that malnutrition and poor oral health in children, older adults are prone to the development of oral disease. Malnutrition has multiple effects on oral cavity with subsequent development of oral disease. Altered tissue homeostasis, reduced resistance to microbial biofilms and tissue repair capacity are result of malnutrition. It is associated with salivary gland changes, enamel hypoplasia and dental caries. Change in the salivary characteristics reduces the defense mechanism of saliva and its ability to buffer the plaque acids [29].

5. Conclusion

Various studies have shown that malnutrition and protein-energy malnutrition affects tooth eruption patterns, enamel hypoplasia, dental caries prevalence, and periodontal ligament. They also have other effects on the oral cavity, like inflammation of the lining of the oral cavity, salivary gland hypofunction, the tongue, and oral ulcers. Malnutrition is a risk to oral health and poor oral health, in turn, leads to malnutrition with unfavorable socio-demographic factors, which calls for a need to improve the living conditions and adequate utilization of available health and nutritional supplementary services through an intersectoral approach.

Conflicts of interest

The authors of this manuscript declare that they have no conflicts of interest, real or perceived, financial or non-financial in this article.

Author details

Kempaiah Siddaiah Madhusudhan[1*] and M.R. Pallavi[2]

1 Department of Pediatric and Preventive Dentistry, The Oxford Dental College, Bengaluru, India

2 Department of Biochemistry, MMK and SDM Mahila Maha Vidyalaya, Mysore, India

*Address all correspondence to: sudhannks@gmail.com

References

[1] Psoter WJ, Reid BC, Katz RV. Malnutrition and dental caries: A review of the literature. Caries Research. 2005;**39**(6):441-447. DOI: 10.1159/000088178 PMID: 16251787; PMCID: PMC1362953

[2] Russell SL, Psoter WJ, Jean-Charles G, Prophte S, Gebrian B. Protein-energy malnutrition during early childhood and periodontal disease in the permanent dentition of Haitian adolescents aged 12-19 years: A retrospective cohort study. International Journal of Paediatric Dentistry. 2010;**20**(3):222-229. DOI: 10.1111/j.1365-263X.2010.01031.x PMID: 20409204; PMCID: PMC2866123

[3] Sheetal A, Hiremath VK, Patil AG, Sajjansetty S, Kumar SR. Malnutrition and its oral outcome - a review. Journal of Clinical and Diagnostic Research. 2013;**7**(1):178-180. DOI: 10.7860/JCDR/2012/5104.2702 PMID: 23449967; PMCID: PMC3576783

[4] Girish Babu KL, Subramaniam P, Madhusudan KS. Association of nutritional status and dental health among 3 - 6 -year-old children of a south Indian population. Saudi Journal of Oral Sciences. 2019;**6**:31-36

[5] Griffin SO, Jones JA, Brunson D, Griffin PM, Bailey WD. Burden of oral disease among older adults and implications for public health priorities. American Journal of Public Health. 2012;**102**(3):411-418. DOI: 10.2105/AJPH.2011.300362 PMID: 22390504; PMCID: PMC3487659

[6] Association of State and Territorial Dental Directors (ASTDD) Best Practices Committee. Best Practice Approach: Oral Health in the Older Adult Population (Age 65 and Older) [Monograph on the Internet]. Reno, NV: Association of State and Territorial Dental Directors; 2017. 29p Available from: http://www.astdd.org

[7] Ehizele AO, Ojehanon PI, Akhionbare O. Nutrition and Oral health. Journal of Postgraduate Medicine. 2009;**11**(1):76-82

[8] De Onis M, Monteiro C, Clugston G. The Worldwide Magnitude of Protein-Energy Malnutrition: An Overview from the WHO Global Database on Child Growth. 71, no. 6. Geneva, Switzerland: World Health Organization; 1993

[9] Madhusudhan KS, Pallavi MR. Malnutrition-a risk for oral health. International Journal of Science and Research. 2019;**8**(4):74-77

[10] El Hélou M, Boulos C, Adib SM, Tabbal N. Relationship between oral health and nutritional status in the elderly: A pilot study in Lebanon. Journal of Clinical Gerontology and Geriatrics. 2014;**5**(3):91-95

[11] Sheiham A, Steele J. Does the condition of the mouth and teeth affect the ability to eat certain foods, nutrient and dietary intake and nutritional status amongst older people? Public Health Nutrition. 2001;**4**(3):797-803. DOI: 10.1079/phn2000116 PMID: 11415487

[12] Scardina GA, Messina P. Good oral health and diet. Journal of Biomedicine & Biotechnology. 2012;**2012**:720692. DOI: 10.1155/2012/720692 PMID: 22363174; PMCID: PMC3272860

[13] Moynihan P, Petersen PE. Diet, nutrition and the prevention of dental diseases. Public Health Nutrition. 2004;**7**(1A):201-226

[14] Field EA, Speechley JA, Rugman FR, Varga E, Tyldesley WR. Oral signs and symptoms in patients with undiagnosed vitamin B12 deficiency. Journal of Oral Pathology & Medicine. 1995;**24**(10):468-470. DOI: 10.1111/j.1600-0714.1995.tb01136.x PMID: 8600284

[15] Psoter WJ, Spielman AL, Gebrian B, St Jean R, Katz RV. Effect of childhood malnutrition on salivary flow and pH. Archives of Oral Biology. 2008;**53**(3):231-237. DOI: 10.1016/j.archoralbio.2007.09.007 PMID: 17983611; PMCID: PMC2268214

[16] Psoter W, Gebrian B, Prophete S, Reid B, Katz R. Effect of early childhood malnutrition on tooth eruption in Haitian adolescents. Community Dentistry and Oral Epidemiology. 2008;**36**(2):179-189. DOI: 10.1111/j.1600-0528.2007.00386.x PMID: 18333882

[17] Thomaz EB, Cangussu MC, da Silva AA, Assis AM. Is malnutrition associated with crowding in permanent dentition? International Journal of Environmental Research and Public Health. 2010;**7**(9):3531-3544. DOI: 10.3390/ijerph7093531 PMID: 20948941; PMCID: PMC2954562

[18] Pontes HA, Neto NC, Ferreira KB, Fonseca FP, Vallinoto GM, Pontes FS, et al. Oral manifestations of vitamin B12 deficiency: A case report. Journal of the Canadian Dental Association. 2009;**75**(7):533-537 PMID: 19744365

[19] Kozlak ST, Walsh SJ, Lalla RV. Reduced dietary intake of vitamin B12 and folate in patients with recurrent aphthous stomatitis. Journal of Oral Pathology & Medicine. 2010;**39**(5):420-423. DOI: 10.1111/j.1600-0714.2009.00867.x PMID: 20141576; PMCID: PMC3323114

[20] Rugg-Gunn AJ, Nunn JH. Nutrition, Diet, and Oral Health. USA: Oxford University Press; 1999

[21] Johansson I, Lenander-Lumikari M, Saellström AK. Saliva composition in Indian children with chronic protein-energy malnutrition. Journal of Dental Research. 1994;**73**(1):11-19

[22] Alvarez J, Lewis CA, Saman C, Caceda J, Montalvo J, Figueroa ML, et al. Chronic malnutrition, dental caries, and tooth exfoliation in Peruvian children aged 3-9 years. The American Journal of Clinical Nutrition. 1988;**48**(2):368-372

[23] Alvarez JO. Nutrition, tooth development, and dental caries. The American Journal of Clinical Nutrition. 1995;**61**(2):410S-416S

[24] Hildebolt CF. Effect of vitamin D and calcium on periodontitis. Journal of Periodontology. 2005;**76**(9):1576-1587

[25] Touyz LZ. Vitamin C, oral scurvy and periodontal disease. South African Medical Journal. 1984;**65**(21):838-842

[26] Burks CE, Jones CW, Braz VA, Swor RA, Richmond NL, Hwang KS, et al. Risk factors for malnutrition among older adults in the emergency department: A multicenter study. Journal of the American Geriatrics Society. 2017;**65**(8):1741-1747

[27] Zelig R, Byham-Gray L, Singer SR, Hoskin ER, Fleisch Marcus A, Verdino G, et al. Dentition and malnutrition risk in community-dwelling older adults. The Journal of Aging Research and Clinical Practice. 2018;7:107-104

[28] Mathad V, Shivprasad S. Malnutrition: A daunting problem for India's spectacular growth.

Indian Journal of Clinical Practice. 2013;**23**(11):760-764

[29] Madhusudhan KS, Khargekar N. Nutritional status and its relationship with dental caries among 3-6-year-old Anganwadi children. International Journal of Clinical Pediatric Dentistry. 2020;**13**(1):6-10

Section 4

Dental Materials

Chapter 5

Role of Metals in Pediatric Oral Health

Shubha Joshi, Pronob Sanyal and Jyotsna Arun Patil

Abstract

Prefabricated stainless steel crowns (SSCs) are the regular dental prosthesis cemented to primary molars in children. Previously used SSC, which contained up to 72% nickel, is associated with nickel sensitivity. Hence, the new generation of SSC that contains only 9–12% nickel was developed. Stainless steel orthodontic materials and stainless steel crowns (SSC) are the two major devices in pediatric patients that contain heavy metals. Measurable amounts of nickel and chromium in the saliva and serum are released from this prosthesis without reaching toxic levels. Allergic reaction in a form of gingivitis was reported after 3 months in 20% of the females and 10% of the males, and it disappeared a month after appliance removal. Several studies reported that there is more leaching of metals in acidic pH. Many different types of alloys are now available in the market to be used for dental restorations and fixed prostheses, and the rates of metal leaching from these alloys are not known. The common criterion for all these fixed prosthodontic materials is their permanent existence in the oral cavity for a prolonged time without the ability to be removed by the patient. Let us know these elements in detail in this chapter.

Keywords: base metal alloys, prefabricated stainless steel alloys, allergy, crowns, pediatric oral health

1. Introduction

Earlier, the precious metals such as silver and gold were commonly used for dental restoration. However, since 20th century, use of noble metals for dental prosthesis has reduced due to their high cost and unavailability; alternative metal alloys of nickel, chromium, cobalt, molybdenum, manganese, iron, copper, and zinc are used more. Numerous researchers have developed new alloys that not only are less expensive than gold but also have properties that are more suitable for specific applications [1–6].

The heavy metals used for dental prosthesis have a greater specific gravity that is five times more than water. Mainly, these heavy metals are found on the earth's outer layer in all ecosystems at varying concentration and occupy groups IIA to VIA in the periodic table [7].

The fabricated prosthesis is made of alloys containing Ni, Co, Cr, and Mo in different percentages. Biodegradation of these alloys occurs due to the different properties of oral environment such as the enzymatic, thermal, and microbiological

[8]. Elements like Ni, Co, and Cr are known to be cytogenic, mutagenic, and allergenic [9]. The most common causes of metal-induced allergic contact dermatitis are Ni and Cr [10].

In oral atmosphere, metal crowns, PFM crowns, post and core, prefabricated crowns, orthodontic brackets, and implants are continuously exposed to different conditions such as temperature, mechanical fatigue, acidic pH, and susceptibility of alloy to corrosion [11]. It is well-known from the literature that leaching of heavy metals from dental restorations occurs in saliva.

Different types of dental casting alloys are now available in the market, which mainly consist of Ni, Cr, Co, and Mo and are being used for several years in dental restorations. Leaching of these heavy metals from dental casting alloys in saliva is well documented in literature, which are absorbed across the GIT, leading to increase blood levels and then may affect the vital organs such as liver, kidney, and lung. Leaching of heavy metals from dental casting alloys is affected by various factors such as pH, duration of prosthesis used, protein-rich solution, masticatory load, wear, and diet. Acidic pH, prolonged use of prosthesis, protein-rich solution, and heavy masticatory load are directly proportional to the release of heavy metals from dental casting alloy (DCA).

2. Use of metals in pediatric oral health

Stainless steel orthodontic materials, space maintainers, and stainless steel crowns (SSC) are the major devices used in pediatric patients that contain heavy metals. In pedodontics, the prefabricated stainless steel crowns have been preferred for deciduous dentition and used temporarily for 3–4 years over the prepared tooth since ages on a deciduous tooth till the tooth is extracted or exfoliated. These are available in assorted packs of different dimensions.

Prefabricated stainless steel crowns (SSCs) are the regular dental prosthesis cemented to primary molars in children. Previously used SSC that contained up to 72% nickel is associated with nickel sensitivity [12]. Hence, the new generation of SSC that contains only 9–12% nickel was developed [13]. All these alloys have to tolerate pH from food and plaque, tooth brushing condition, and the heavy masticatory load. Wear is a key factor that can accelerate corrosive processes in vivo. It is expected that the effect of element release will have to be understood for selecting different kinds of alloys for the purpose of dental restorations. Measurable amounts of nickel and chromium in the saliva and serum were seen to be released from these prosthesis without reaching toxic levels [14]. The release from these appliances showed an increase over the first week after placement and then decreased over time [15]. Allergic reaction in the form of gingivitis was seen after 3 months in 20% of the females and 10% of the males, and it disappeared a month after appliance removal [16].

3. Alloy composition and properties

Dental alloys are described by their composition that is usually expressed as weight percentage and atomic percentage and by their phase structure (microstructure), which can be either single-phase alloys or multiple-phase alloys. Single-phase alloys have a similar composition throughout their structure, but multiple-phase alloys are not homogenous throughout their structure. The elemental release depends on the interactions between the phase structure and the biologic environment [17]. The elemental release may be caused by a change in surface composition of the alloys. The nickel–chromium alloy, which is a multiphase alloy, is prone to higher corrosion rates, due to the galvanic effects between the microscopic areas of different compositions [18]. It has been shown that there was an alteration in cellular function due to ions released from Ni-Cr alloys [19].

The alloy reactivity is governed by thermodynamic principles and electrochemical reaction kinetics, where the alloy will either remain stable in its elemental form or oxidize into its ionic form (corrosion) Nickel–chromium alloys are not thermodynamically stable, and their corrosion resistance depends on the formation of the thin oxide layer [20].

4. Functions of alloying elements

Cobalt: It adds strength, rigidity, and hardness to the alloy. It has a high melting point.

Chromium: The passivating result of chromium ensures corrosion resistance. The amount of chromium is directly proportional to tarnish and corrosion resistance. It reduces the melting point. Chromium with the other elements acts as a hardener. 30% chromium is thought to be the maximum for gaining mechanical properties.

Nickel: Nickel and cobalt are exchangeable. It decreases hardness, strength, fusion temperature, and modulus of elasticity. It improves ductility.

Molybdenum or tungsten: They improve the hardness. Molybdenum is chosen over tungsten as it reduces ductility and also refines grain structure.

Iron, copper: These are principally hardeners.

Beryllium: It reduces fusion temperature and refines grain structure.

Manganese and silicon: During melting, these help to avoid the oxidation of other elements. They are also hardeners.

Boron: It reduces ductility and acts as a deoxidizer and hardener.

Carbon: Small amount of carbides formed by the carbon with any of the metallic constituents improves the strength of the alloy, but excess carbide will increase the brittleness. Thus, control of carbon content in the alloy is important [21–23].

5. Elemental release

The factors that affect the elemental release from the alloy are many such as alloy composition, multiple phases, chemical character of the corrosive medium, exposure time, and temperature. There are many studies to assess the release of elements from dental casting alloys. The release of elements from dental casting alloys has been investigated by many different researchers using different materials and methods [24–33]. It is proven that at certain environmental conditions, the release of elements from the alloy is affected. Cell culture or different solutions such as normal saline, bovine serum solution, artificial saliva, tissue culture media, and diluted acids are used to evaluate the corrosion [24, 26, 29]. Leaching is tested in different mouthwashes and also in different pH solutions. An alcohol-based mouthwash resulted in the release of the highest amounts of Ni and Cr ions due to its lower pH.

5.1 Methods of testing elemental release

The elemental release can be measured by atomic absorption spectroscopy (AAS), inductively coupled plasma-atomic emission spectrometry (ICP-AES), or inductively coupled plasma mass spectrometry (ICP-MS) in different environments. AAS has been used with cell culture medium [34, 35], pH 7 phosphate buffer solution or saline, saline with 3% bovine serum albumin, and 3% serum [35]. ICP-MS was used for samples of artificial oral saliva [36]; ICP-AES was used for samples of artificial oral saliva, cell culture medium, and acidic pH [37, 38].

5.2 Effects of pH

The interest in studying elemental release is mainly due its relationship to the biocompatibility of the alloy. Elemental release has been reported for base metal alloys [39, 40] and for other types of alloys and solders [41–43], which focuses on the measurement of release during the exposure to a biologic medium or artificial saliva at different durations. The effect of a steady reduced pH on the elemental release from Ni-based alloys has been reported to increase Ni release [29, 40]. In the oral cavity, alloys may be exposed to transient pH changes either from foods or from plaque [44].

5.3 Effects of proteins

Behavior of proteins to the corrosion reactions could in 2 ways: Proteins bind to metal ions and move them far from the interface, thus aiding further dissolution, or these proteins could be engaged to the surface of the metal and obstruct the diffusion of oxygen, making it difficult to repassivate the surface.

5.4 Effects of saliva

The composition and properties of saliva may be affected by many physiological variables such as nutrition, diet, and salivary flow [45, 46]. According to Edgar and O'Mullane [47], hormones, drugs, and various diseases also influence saliva composition. Wirz et al. [48] and Grahmmer reported saliva samples of the control group without any metal restorations to contain the metals Ag, Cr, Cu, Fe, Ni, and Zn.

5.5 Effects of duration

The elemental release has been studied for different durations, and it was reported that the release may change significantly with time for some formulations over 80 h [49], and by 10 months, the release reduced lower than in the initial weeks and was constant after 100 days of exposure [28].

With the evaluation of cytotoxicity of nickel-chromium alloys after prolonged conditioning (168 h), it was found that alloy toxicity varied with the conditioning solution. The saline/BSA conditioning solution reduced the cytotoxicity of the alloys compared with unconditioned alloy cytotoxicity [50].

6. Nickel

6.1 Properties of nickel

6.1.1 Daily requirements of nickel

A daily dose of 0.001–0.0024 mg/kg/day can be estimated using a reference body weight of 70 kg (**Figure 1**) [51].

6.1.2 Sources of nickel

Nickel is widely distributed in the environment and can be found in air, water, and soil [52, 53]. Dusts from volcanic emissions and the weathering of rocks and soils are the usual sources of atmospheric nickel. The level of Ni in ambient air is minute as 6–20 ng·m-3, but in air contaminated by anthropogenic sources, it may increase to 150 ng Ni·m-3. Ni in uncontaminated water is around 300 ng Ni·dm-3. Farm soil contains approximately 3–1000 mg $Ni{\cdot}kg^{-1}$ soil, but in the soil near metal refineries and dried sludge, the Ni concentration can reach up to 24,000–53,000 mg $Ni{\cdot}kg^{-1}$. Ni compounds in soil at pH < 6.5 are relatively soluble, but at pH > 6.7, they are insoluble hydroxides [54–56].

6.1.3 Nickel exposure

The primary reason for Ni exposure is inhalation followed by ingestion and dermal contact. This happens in Ni and its alloy industries or during welding and electroplating. Nickel industries show up to 1 $mg{\cdot}m^{-3}$ of nickel. The advent of new technologies has reduced these exposures [57, 58]. Inhalation is the primary route of occupational exposure, and it elevates the Ni levels in blood, urine, and body tissues.

6.1.4 Absorption of nickel

Nickel acts as a cofactor in the absorption of iron from the intestine. Also, Ni may be absorbed as the soluble nickel ion and soluble nickel compounds may be

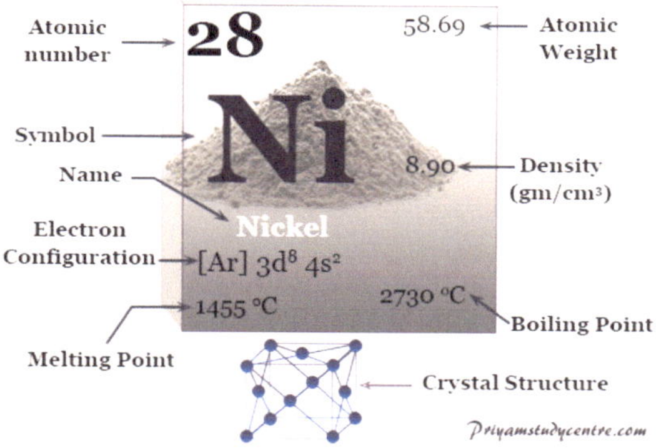

Figure 1.
Properties of nickel. Source: https://www.priyamstudycentre.com/2021/01/nickel.html.

phagocytized. The extent of absorption of Ni in the lungs depends on its chemical form and deposition site and also determined by the size, shape, density, and electrical charge [51, 59]. The mucociliary transport of the respiratory tract removes portions of Ni, which results in the material entering the GIT. Ni is inadequately absorbed from the GIT, but exposure from diet and drinking water provides most of the intake of nickel and nickel compounds [60, 61]. Dermal absorption of Ni is poor, but its compounds like nickel chloride or nickel sulfate can penetrate the skin. Pharmacokinetic studies indicate that nickel is absorbed through the lungs [62–64], GIT [65–67], and skin [68, 69]. Following absorption from the lungs and the GIT, nickel is excreted in the urine [70–72].

6.1.5 Metabolism of nickel

Nickel metabolism approximately occurs by binding to form ligands and its transport throughout the body. The chemical form of nickel may be altered in the body without being destroyed. Nickel toxicity may be associated with its interference with the physiological processes of manganese, zinc, calcium, and magnesium [61]. Altered transport and serum concentrations of nickel are associated with diseases such as myocardial infarction and acute stroke and burn injury (**Figure 2**) [59].

6.1.6 Excretion of nickel

Most of the ingested Ni is not absorbed and is eliminated mostly through feces. The Ni absorbed from the GIT is excreted in the urine and is mainly associated with low molecular weight complexes that contain amino acids. Nickel can also be eliminated through sweat and milk [73].

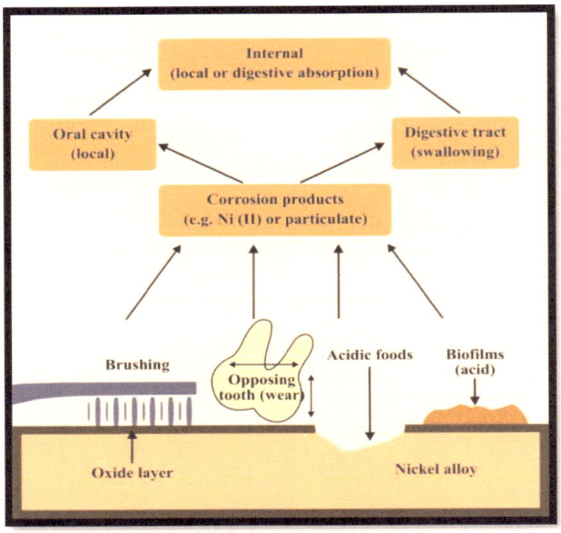

Figure 2.
Corrosion of nickel-based alloys.

6.1.7 Effect on health due to nickel

The toxic effect of Ni is related to the route through which it gets into an organism. Nickel enters the body through inhalation, ingestion, and skin absorption, but the route is determined by its chemical form like the fat soluble Ni carbonyl enters by diffusion or through calcium channels [74], while insoluble nickel particles enter the vertebrate cells by phagocytosis [75]. The main transport protein of nickel in blood is albumin, but nickel can also bind to histidine and α2-macroglobulin [57, 76] and in this form is circulated throughout the tissues. A number of nickel-binding proteins including α1-antitrypsin, α1-lipoprotein, and prealbumin were also described [77]. Nickel is found in high concentrations in bone, brain, respiratory organ, liver excretory organ, and endocrine glands. It is also marked in hair, breast milk, nails, and saliva. It is also proved that Ni was capable of transplacental transfer in rodents. Ni gets excreted through sweat, urine, feces, and bile. It does not get accumulated in the body [78]. The effects of Ni contact manifest as respiratory tract cancers, contact dermatitis, fibrosis of lung, and kidney and cardiovascular diseases [58, 79–81]. Long-term exposure to pollutants of low concentrations leads to chronic effects, and short-term exposure to high concentrations of pollutants leads to acute health effects such as abdominal discomfort, nausea, vomiting, diarrhea, headache, visual disturbance, and cough.

6.2 Chromium

6.2.1 Properties of chromium

6.2.1.1 Daily requirements of chromium

The National Academy of Sciences has established a safe and adequate daily intake for Cr(III) in adults of 50–200 micrograms per day (**Figure 3**) [82].

6.2.2 Sources of chromium

Cr(III) and Cr(VI) are released to the environment from human activities. Coal and oil combustion contributes an estimated 1723 metric tons of chromium per year in atmospheric emissions; however, only 0.2% of this chromium is Cr(VI). In air, Cr(III) does not undergo any reaction, while Cr(VI) reacts with dust particles or other pollutants to form Cr(III). Large amounts of chromium are released in surface waters due to leather tanning, electroplating, and textile industries. The natural source of Cr entry into bodies of water is by leaching from topsoil and rocks. Improperly disposed solid wastes from chromate-processing amenities can be sources of contamination for groundwater, where the chromium dwelling time might be several years. Wind erosion of the soil also makes settled particles airborne, which increases the opportunity for inhalation of chromium. Cr compounds leached by rainwater also migrate through cracks in soil, blacktop roadways, and masonry walls, forming high-content Cr crystals on their surfaces [82].

6.2.3 Exposure of chromium

Inhalation, ingestion, and dermal absorption are the means for Cr to enter the human body. Inhalation and dermal contact are the major causes for occupational

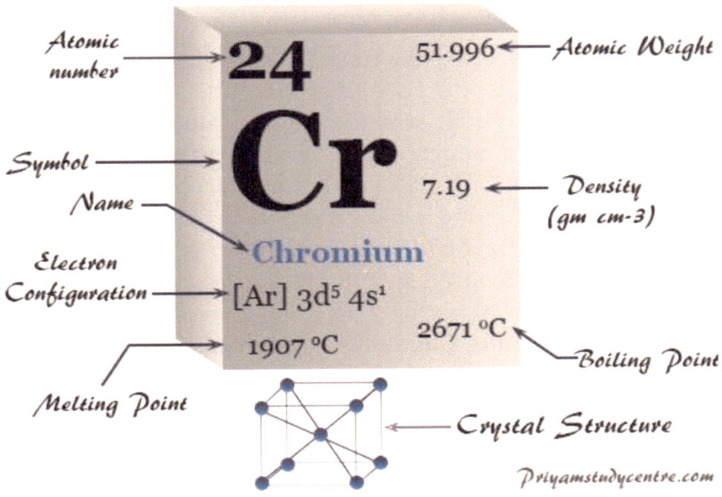

Figure 3.
Properties of chromium. Source: https://www.priyamstudycentre.com/2020/12/chromium.html.

exposure, while ingestion is the main source of exposure through food and water for the general population [54]. Studies have shown increased urinary concentrations of chromium after exposure to Cr(III) by inhalation, indicating respiratory absorption [83–85].

In ingestion of Cr(VI) compounds, they are better absorbed through the intestinal mucosa than the Cr(III) compounds. However, due to the actions of acids in the stomach and other components within the GIT, most of an ingested Cr(VI) dosage is converted to Cr(III) [86]. There is evidence from occupational studies that absorption of Cr(VI) compounds can occur through intact skin [87].

6.2.4 Absorption of chromium

The rate of Cr absorption from the GIT is moderately low and depends on factors like valence state where Cr[VI] is more easily absorbed than Cr[III], the chemical form where organic chromium is more easily absorbed than inorganic chromium, the water solubility of the compound, and gastrointestinal transit time. Absorption of Cr(VI) occurs rapidly through erythrocytes and is reduced to Cr(III) inside the red blood cells. On the contrary, Cr(III) binds directly to transferrin, an iron-transporting protein in the plasma, without crossing red blood cell membranes [82, 85, 88].

6.2.5 Metabolism of chromium

Glutathione reduces Cr(VI) in the RBC into Cr(III), which gets trapped in the RBC as the membrane is not permeable. Ultimately, the diffusion of Cr(VI), the reduction to Cr(III), and the complexing to nucleic acids and proteins within the cell will cause the concentration equilibrium to change [82]. Extracellular reduction of Cr(VI) to

Cr(III) reduces the toxicity. The difference between the extracellular Cr(VI) and intracellular Cr(III) dictates the amount of toxic effects [86].

In spite of the source, Cr(III) is present in the body in plasma or tissues. Lungs, spleen, bone marrow, kidney, liver, and lymph nodes take up the greatest amount of Cr(III) as a protein complex.

6.2.6 Excretion of chromium

Absorbed chromium is excreted primarily as urine. Within 8 hours of ingestion, the kidney excretes about 60% of absorbed Cr(VI) in the form of Cr(III), and around 10% is eliminated by biliary excretion. Also, small amounts of Cr are excreted through sweat, nails, milk, and hair (**Figure 4**) [82, 89].

6.2.7 Effects on health due to chromium

Chromium compounds are respiratory tract irritants and can cause pulmonary sensitization. Chronic inhalation of Cr(VI) compounds increases the risk of lung, nasal, and sinus cancer [90]. Contact with Cr(VI) compounds can cause severe dermatitis and usually painless skin ulcers [91, 92]. Cr(VI) is recognized as a human carcinogen. Reversible renal tubular damage can occur after low-dose, chronic Cr(VI) exposure [93]. Cr(VI) compounds can cause mild to severe liver abnormalities. Some Cr(VI) compounds, such as potassium dichromate and chromium trioxide, are caustic and irritating to the gastrointestinal mucosal tissue.

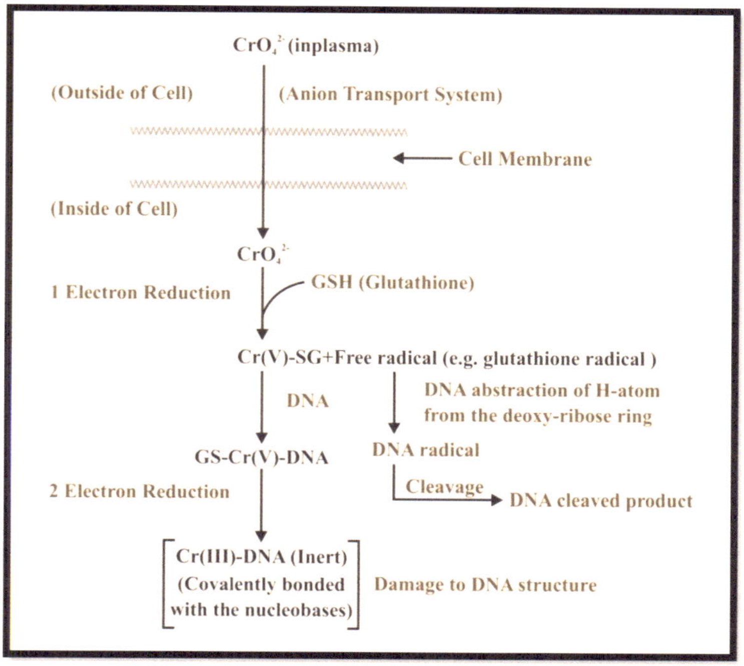

Figure 4.
Schematic representation of uptake reduction model.

6.3 Cobalt

6.3.1 Properties of cobalt

6.3.1.1 Daily requirements of cobalt

As a component of cyanocobalmin (vitamin B12), cobalt is essential in the body; the Recommended Dietary Allowance of vitamin B12 is 2.4 μg/day, which contains 0.1 μg of cobalt (**Figure 5**) [94].

6.3.2 Sources of cobalt

Cobalt is naturally available in water, soil, rock, plants, and air. Also, it may settle on land from forest fires, seawater spray, volcanic eruptions, and windblown dust. It can again get into surface water due to leaching and overflow by rainwater wash. High concentrations of cobalt are seen in phosphate rocks, soil near ore deposits, and soils contaminated by traffic, industrial pollution. Coal-fired power plants and incinerators, vehicular exhaust, mining and processing of cobalt-containing ores, and the production and use of cobalt alloys and chemicals also release small amounts of cobalt [94].

6.3.3 Exposure to cobalt

Cobalt is widely dispersed in the environment in low concentrations. One can be exposed to small amounts of cobalt by breathing air, drinking water, and eating food containing it. Food is the largest source of cobalt intake; about 11 micrograms of cobalt is consumed in a day [95].

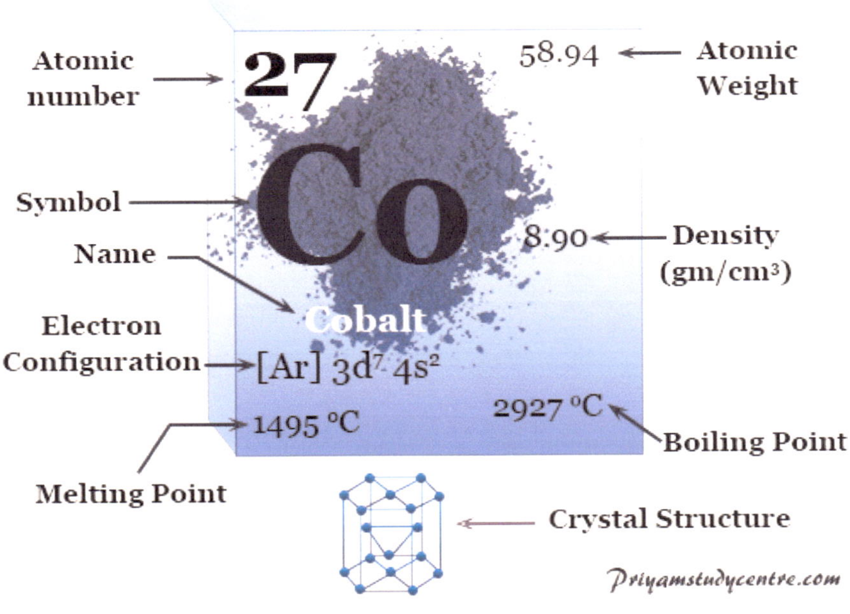

Figure 5.
Properties of cobalt. Source: https://www.priyamstudycentre.com/2021/01/cobalt.html.

6.3.4 Absorption of cobalt

Cobalt compounds deposit in the lungs after inhalation exposure based on their aerosol characteristics. Cobalt particles that are physiologically insoluble are removed by phagocytosis and/or mucociliary transport [96]. Soluble forms of cobalt enter the bloodstream through the alveolar or bronchial walls. Nutritional status also is an important factor in cobalt absorption due to oral exposure, with both overnight fasting and iron deficiency resulting in increased cobalt absorption [97, 98]. It is also found that Co and Fe share a common absorptive pathway in the intestines, though cobalt absorption takes place without ferritin.

6.3.5 Metabolism of cobalt

Cobalt is essential in the body because it is a component of cyanocobalamin (Vit B12) [99], which is also involved in hematopoiesis; deficiency of this leads to pernicious anemia (**Figure 6**) [100].

6.3.6 Excretion of cobalt

Presently, there are no available data on the excretion of soluble cobalt particles in humans. Following an exposure to insoluble cobalt compounds (cobalt metal, cobalt oxides), elimination from the body appears to follow three-phase kinetics (**Table 1**).

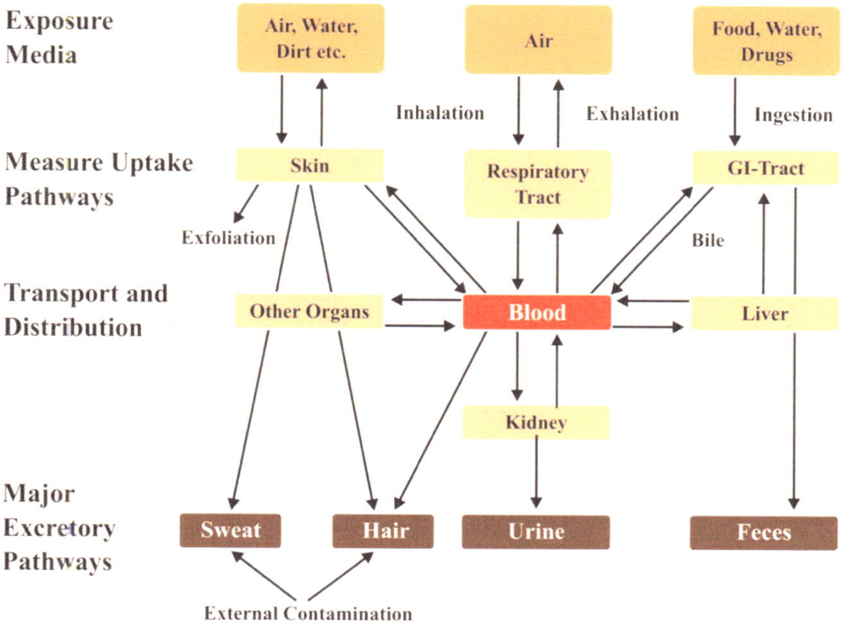

Figure 6.
Metabolism after exposure to heavy metals.

Kinetics	Clearance
First phase [101, 102]	Mucociliary clearance of particles deposited in the tracheobronchial region. *Half-time* on the order of **2–44 hours**
Second phase [103, 104]	Macrophag mediated clearance from the lung. *Half-time* on the order of **10–78 days**
Third phase [103–106]	long-term clearance from the lungs. *Half-time* on the order of years

Table 1.
List of different phases of kinetics in cobalt excretion.

6.3.7 Effect on health due to cobalt

Cobalt has both beneficial and harmful effects on human health. Cobalt is beneficial for humans because it is a part of vitamin B1. 0.16–1.0 mg cobalt/kg of body weight has been used as a treatment for anemia, including in pregnant women, as it causes production of RBCs. Exposure to 0.005 mg cobalt/m3 causes effects on the lungs, including asthma, pneumonia, and wheezing [106]. People exposed to 0.007 mg cobalt/m3 at work have also developed allergies to cobalt that have resulted in asthma and skin rashes [107].

6.4 Molybdenum

6.4.1 Properties of molybdenum

6.4.1.1 Daily requirement of molybdenum

Molybdenum is an essential nutrient; the nutritional requirement for adults is 45 μg/day (0.64 μg/kg/day) (**Figure** 7) [108, 109].

6.4.2 Sources of molybdenum

Molybdenum is found in higher concentrations in air, water, and soil. Molybdenum concentrations in ambient air have been reported to range from below detection limits to 0.03 mg/m^3 [110].

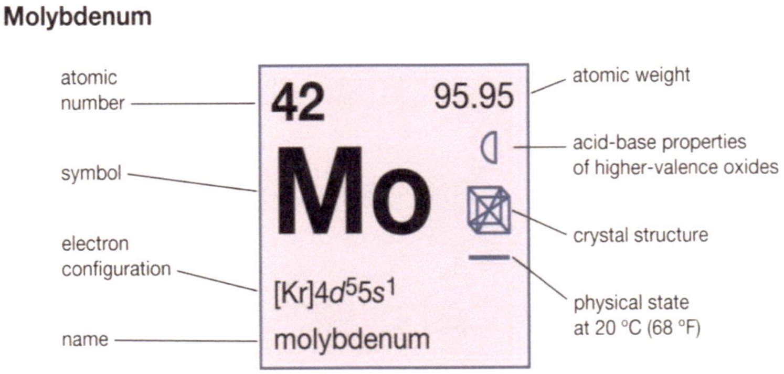

Figure 7.
Properties of molybdenum. Source: https://www.priyamstudycentre.com/2021/01/molybdenum.html, https://www.google.com/url?sa=i&url=https%3A%2F%2Fwww.britannica.com%2Fscience%2Fmolybdenum&psig=AOvVaw36J2pmNBtTjQzFFaxoVK7I&ust=1675683204305000&source=images&cd=vfe&ved=2ahUKEwjc37rCpP78AhVyC7cAHSoEAikQr4kDegUIARDeAQ

6.4.3 Exposure to molybdenum

The general population's exposure to molybdenum is almost entirely through food. Rich sources of molybdenum are found in beans, cereal grains, leafy vegetables, legumes, liver, and milk [111]. Molybdenum contamination of drinking water is seen due to influence of industrial effluents (**Figure 8**).

6.4.4 Absorption of molybdenum

Inhaled molybdenum particles are distributed via (1) bronchial and tracheal mucociliary transport to the gastrointestinal tract; (2) transport to thoracic lymph nodes; or (3) absorption into blood and/or lymph and transfer to other tissues. Particles are cleared from the pulmonary region primarily by absorption, lymph drainage, macrophage phagocytosis and migration, and upward mucociliary flow. Dissolved molybdenum is absorbed into the blood. The rate of absorption depends on solubility. Ingested molybdenum that is absorbed depends on numerous factors, including molybdenum dose level, fasting, diet, and nutritional status [112, 113].

6.4.5 Metabolism of molybdenum

Molybdenum exists in several valence states and may undergo oxidation and reduction. The primary form of molybdenum that interacts with enzyme systems is MoVI, as the molybdate anion (MoVIO22-) [114]. After molybdate is taken into a cell, it is incorporated into a molybdopterin to form molybdenum cofactor (Moco). Moco is a sulfur-molybdate complex that forms the prosthetic group in molybdenum-dependent enzymes [115, 116]. Moco is extremely sensitive to oxidation, and it binds

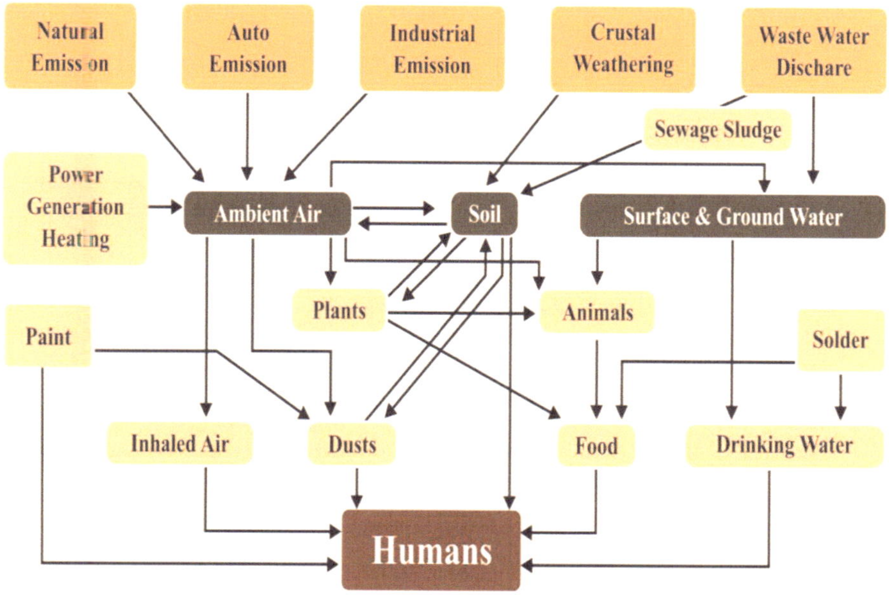

Figure 8.
Pathways of human exposure to heavy metals [ATSDR 2005].

to a Moco-binding protein in the cell (Mendel and Kruse 2012) where it is stored to meet the cell's demand for molybdenum enzymes. Molybdate forms complexes with copper and binds to plasma proteins as a copper-molybdenum-sulfur (Cu-Mo-S) complex [117, 118].

6.4.6 *Excretion of molybdenum*

Absorbed molybdenum is excreted as urine and feces in humans. Urine is the dominant excretion route, accounting for the excretion of approximately 75–90% of the absorbed dose [119, 120].

6.4.7 *Effects on health due to molybdenum*

Tetrathiomolybdate forms a tripartite complex with copper and protein and prevents copper absorption through the gastrointestinal tract [121]; thus, tetrathiomolybdate is used in the treatment of Wilson's disease. Significant increases in serum and urine copper levels were observed in men exposed to 0.022 mg molybdenum/kg/day for 10 days, as compared to exposure to 0.00771 mg molybdenum/kg/day for 10 days [122]. However, there was no difference in fecal excretion of copper, suggesting that copper absorption was not affected. In contrast, another study [123] showed no significant changes in serum copper levels when exposed to molybdenum levels of 22–1490 μg/day (0.0003–0.02 mg/kg/day) for 24 days (**Table 2**).

Sr. No.	References	Study hypothesis	Research finding
1	Ros C. Randall et al. [13]	To carry out an extensive literature review of the use and efficiency of preformed metal crowns for primary and permanent molar teeth.	PMCs are superior to amalgam restorations for multi-surface cavities in primary molar teeth.
2	Bhaskar V et al. [124]	To evaluate *in vitro* biodegradation of space maintainers made of two different company bands (Dantaurum, Unitek) using atomic adsorption spectrophotometer.	Ni ranging from 4.95 to 7.78 ppm and chromium from 1.70 to 4.54 ppm were released through an artificial salivary medium. Release of Ni and Cr reached a peak level on the 7th day, then decreased with time.
3	David Keinan et al. [125]	To analyze the absorption of metal ions released from stainless-steel crowns by root surface of primary molars.	Stainless-steel crowns release nickel, chromium, and iron in the oral environment, and the ions are absorbed by the primary molar roots.
4	Hiroe Kodaira et al. [126]	To assess alterations in levels of iron, chromium, and nickel released from preformed crowns and compare these levels with standard values.	Accumulation of trace elements released from preformed crowns used in restoration of primary teeth (3 M stainless-steel primary molar crowns) does not affect the body.
5	Kulkarni P et al. [127]	To measure the Ni ion release from conventionally preformed stainless-steel crowns (SSCs), and to determine the maximum no of appliances that can be given to an individual without reaching toxic levels.	The release of nickel and chromium was very much below when compared with the average dietary intake of nickel (200–300 ppm/day), which was not capable of causing any toxic effects.

Sr. No.	References	Study hypothesis	Research finding
6	Leila Basir et al. [128]	To evaluate the effect of pH, time, oral temperature, and SSCs' trimming on the nickel releasing.	The concentration of released nickel decreased with trimming of margins and increased when temperature increased. Time and pH had no significant effect on released nickel.

Table 2.
List of previous literature related to different pre-fabricated crowns.

Author details

Shubha Joshi[1]*, Pronob Sanyal[1] and Jyotsna Arun Patil[2]

1 Department of Prosthodontics and Crown and Bridge, School of Dental Sciences, Krishna Vishwa Vidyapeeth, Karad, Maharashtra, India

2 Department of Biochemistry, Krishna Vishwa Vidyapeeth, Karad, Maharashtra, India

*Address all correspondence to: drkamnoorshubha@gmail.com

References

[1] Ring ME. A thousand years of dental implants: A definitive history part 1. The Compendium of Continuing Education in Dentistry. 1995;**16**:1060-1064

[2] Kusy RP. Orthodontic biomaterials: From the past to the present. The Angle Orthodontist. 2002;**72**:501-512

[3] Leinfelder KF. An evaluation of casting alloys used for restorative procedures. Journal of the American Dental Association (1939). 1997;**128**: 37-45

[4] Morris HF, Manz M, Stoffer W, Weir D. Casting alloys: The materials and "the clinical effects". Advances in Dental Research. 1992;**6**:28-31

[5] Paffenbarger GC, Caul HJ, Dickson MA. Base metal alloys for oral restorations. Journal of the American Dental Association (1939). 1943;**30**: 852-862

[6] Roach M. Base metal alloys used for dental restorations and implants. Dental Clinics of North America. 2007;**51**: 603-627

[7] Das KK, Chandramouli Reddy R, Bagoji IB, Das S, Bagali SL, Mullur L, et al. Primary concept of nickel toxicity – An overview. Journal of Basic and Clinical Physiology and Pharmacology. 2019;**30**(2):141-152

[8] Das KK, Reddy RC, Bagoji IB, Das S, Bagali S, Mullur L, et al. Primary concept of nickel toxicity - an overview. Journal of Basic and Clinical Physiology and Pharmacology. 2018;**30**:141-152

[9] Holm C, Morisbak E, Kalfoss T, Dahl JE. In vitro element release and biological aspects of base-metal alloys for metal-ceramic applications. Acta Biomaterialia Odontologica Scandinavica. 2015;**1**:70-75

[10] Denizoglu S, Duymus ZY. Evaluation of cobalt, chromium, and nickel concentrations in plasma and blood of patients with removable partial dentures. Dental Materials Journal. 2006;**25**:365-370

[11] Efeoglu N, Ozturk B, Coker C, Cotert S, Bulbul M. In vitro release of elements from prosthodontic base metal alloys: Effect of protein-containing biologic environments. The International Journal of Prosthodontics. 2006;**19**: 250-252

[12] Feasby WH, Ecclestone ER, Grainger RM. Nickel sensitivity in pediatric dental patients. Pediatric Dentistry. 1988;**10**(2):127-129

[13] Ros C. Randall, preformed metal crowns for primary and permanent molar teeth: Review of the literature. Pediatric Dentistry. 2002;**24**:489-500

[14] Agaoglu G, Arun T, Izgu B, Yarat A. Nickel and chromium levels in the saliva and serum of patients with fixed orthodontic appliances. Angle Orthodontist. 2001;**71**(5):375-379

[15] Barrett RD, Bishara SE, Quinn JK. Biodegradation of orthodontic appliances. Part I. biodegradation of nickel and chromium in vitro. American Journal of Orthodontics and Dentofacial Orthopedics. 1993;**103**(1):8-14

[16] Jensen CS, Lisby S, Baadsgaard O, Vølund A, Menne T. Decrease in nickel sensitization in a Danish schoolgirl population with ears pierced after implementation of a nickelexposure regulation. British Journal of Dermatology. 2002;**146**(4):636-642

[17] Wataha JC. Biocompatibility of dental casting alloys: A review. The Journal of Prosthetic Dentistry. 2000;**83**: 223-234

[18] Wataha JC. Alloys for prosthodontic restorations. The Journal of Prosthetic Dentistry. 2002;**87**:351-363

[19] Messer RLW, Lucas LC. Cytotoxicity of nickel–chromium alloys: Bulk alloys compared to multiple ion salt solutions. Dental Materials. 2000;**16**: 207-212

[20] Lucas LC, Lemons JE. Biodegradation of restorative metallic systems. Advances in Dental Research. 1992;**6**:32e7

[21] Vineeth G, Alla RK, Srinivasa Raju D, Suresh Sajjan MC, Ramaraju AV, Yeleti H. Casting alloys: The saga of their existence and the recipe of their blend. International Journal of Dental Materials. 2019;**1**(1):25-35

[22] Anusavice P. Science of Dental Materials. 11th ed. WB Saunders, Philadelphia: Elsevier; 2012

[23] Craig RG, Powers JH. Restorative dental materials. 11th ed. Mosby, St. Louis: Mosby; 2002

[24] Wataha JC, Malcolm CT, Hanks CT. Correlation between cytotoxicity and the element release by dental casting alloys. The International Journal of Prosthodontics. 1995;**8**:9-14

[25] Brune D. Metal release from dental biomaterials. Biomaterials. 1986;**7**: 163-175

[26] Geis-Gerstorfer JG, Sauer KH, Passler K. Ion release for Ni-Cr-Mo and Co-Cr-Mo casting alloys. The International Journal of Prosthodontics. 1991;**4**:152-158

[27] Tai Y, De Long R, Goodkind RJ, Douglas WH. Leaching of nickel, chromium and beryllium ions from base metal alloy in an artificial oral environment. The Journal of Prosthetic Dentistry. 1992;**68**:692-697

[28] Wataha JC, Lockwood PE. Release of elements from dental casting alloys into cell- culture medium over 10 months. Dental Materials. 1998;**14**:158-163

[29] Covington JS, Me Bridge MA, Slagle WF, Disney AL. Quantifications of nickel and beryllium leakage from base metal casting alloys. The Journal of Prosthetic Dentistry. 1985;**54**:127-136

[30] Wataha JC, Lockwood PE, Khajotia SS, Turner R. Effect of pH on element release from dental casting alloys. The Journal of Prosthetic Dentistry. 1998;**8**:691-698

[31] Nelson SK, Wataha JC, Neme AML, Cibirka RM, Lockwood PE. Cytotoxicity of dental casting alloys pretreated with biologic solutions. The Journal of Prosthetic Dentistry. 1999;**8**:591-596

[32] Wataha JC, Lockwood PE, Noda M, Nelson SK, Mettenburg DJ. Effect of tooth brushing on the toxicity of casting alloys. The Journal of Prosthetic Dentistry. 2002;**87**:94-98

[33] Can G. The release of elements from dental casting alloy into cell-culture medium and artificial saliva. European Journal of Dentistry. 2007;**2**:86-90

[34] Bumgardner JD, Lucas LC. Cellular response to metallic ions released from nickel– Chromium dental alloys. Journal of Dental Research. 1995;**74**:1521-1527

[35] Wataha JC, Lockwood PE, Mettenburg D, Bouillaguet S. Tooth brushing causes elemental release from

dental casting alloys over extended intervals. Journal of Biomedical Materials Research Part B: Applied Biomaterials. 2003;**65**:180-185

[36] Lopez-Alias JF, Martinez-Gomis J, Anglada JM, Peraire M. Ion release from dental casting alloys as assessed by a continuous flow system: Nutritional and toxicological implications. Dental Materials. 2006;**6**:836-841

[37] Schmalz G, Langer H, Schweikl H. Cytotoxicity of dental alloy extracts and corresponding metal salt solutions. Journal of Dental Research. 1998;**77**: 1772-1778

[38] Elshahawy W. Elemental ion release from four different fixed prosthodontic materials. Dental Materials. 2009;**25**: 976-981

[39] Johansson BI, Lemons JE, Hao SQ. Corrosion of dental copper, nickel, and gold alloys in artificial saliva and saline solutions. Dental Materials. 1989;**5**: 324-328

[40] Gerstorfer JG, Sauer KH, Pässler K. Ion release from Ni-Cr-Mo and Co-Cr-Mo casting alloys. The International Journal of Prosthodontics. 1991;**4**: 152-158

[41] Brune D. Mechanisms and kinetics of metal release from dental alloys. International Endodontic Journal. 1988; **21**:135-142

[42] Bergman M, Ginstrup O. Dissolution rate of cadmium from dental gold solder alloys. Acta Odontologica Scandinavica. 1975;**33**:199-210

[43] Vaidyanathan TK, Prasad A. In vitro corrosion and tarnish characterization of typical dental gold compositions. Journal of Biomedical Materials Research. 1981; **15**:191-201

[44] Aamdal-Scheie A, Luan WM, Dahlén G, Fejerskov O. Plaque pH and microflora of dental plaque on sound and carious root surfaces. Journal of Dental Research. 1996;**75**:1901-1908

[45] Keruso H, Moe G. Hensten-Pettersen a salivary nickel and chromium in subjects with different types of fixed orthodontic appliances. American Journal of Orthodontics and Dentofacial Orthopedics. 1997;**111**:595-598

[46] Pfeiffer P, Schwickerath H. Nickell_slichkeit von Dentallegierungenim Speichel. Deutsche zahnärztliche Zeitschrift. 1990;**45**:492-494

[47] Edgar WM, O'Mullane DM. Saliva and Oral Health. 2nd ed. London: British Dental Journal; 1996

[48] Wirz J, Dillena P, Schmidli F. Metalle im Speichel. Die Quintessenz. 1992;**43**:869-874

[49] Wataha JC, Craig RG, Hanks CT. The effects of cleaning on the kinetics of in vitro metal release from dental casting alloys. Journal of Dental Research. 1992; **71**:1417-1422

[50] Nelson SK, Wataha JC, Lockwood PE. Accelerated toxicity testing of casting alloys and reduction of intraoral release of elements. The Journal of Prosthetic Dentistry. 1999;**81**:715-720

[51] ATSDR (Agency for Toxic Substances and Disease Registry). Toxicological Profile for Nickel. Atlanta, GA, USA: ATSDR/U.S. Public Health Service, ATSDR/TP-88/19; 1988

[52] Cempel M, Nikel G. Nickel: A review of its sources and environmental toxicology. Polish Journal of Environmental Studies. 2006;**15**(3): 375-382

[53] Duda-Chodak A, Baszczyk U. The impact of nickel on human health. Journal of Elementology. 2008;**13**(4): 685-696

[54] Barceloux DG. Nickel. Clinical Toxicology. 1999;**37**(2):239-258

[55] Denkhaus E, Salnikow K. Nickel essentiality, toxicity, and carcinogenicity. Critical Reviews in Oncology and Hematology. 2002;**42**: 35-56

[56] Sutherland JE, Costa M. nickel. In: Sarkar B, editor. In: Heavy Metals in the Environment. New York: Marcel decker Inc.; 2002

[57] Kasprzak KS, Sunderman FW Jr, Salnikow K. Nickel carcinogenesis. Mutation Research. 2003;**533**:67-97

[58] Seilkop SK, Oller AR. Respiratory cancer risks associated with low-level nickel exposure: An integrated assessment based on animal, epidemiological, and mechanistic data. Regulatory Toxicology and Pharmacology. 2003;**37**:173-190

[59] Das KK, Das SN, Dhundasi SA. Nickel, its adverse health effects & oxidative stress. The Indian Journal of Medical Research. 2008;**128**:412-425

[60] Goyer R. Toxic effects of metals. In: Amdur MO, Doull JD, Klaassen CD, editors. Casarett and Doull's Toxicology. 4th ed. New York: Pergamon Press; 1991. pp. 623-680

[61] Coogan TP, Latta DM, Snow ET, Costa M. Toxicity and carcinogenicity of nickel compounds. In: McClellan RO, editor. Critical Reviews in Toxicology. Vol. 19. Boca Raton, FL: CRC Press; 1989. pp. 341-384

[62] Bennett BG. Environmental nickel pathways in man. In: Sunderman FW Jr, editor. Nickel in the Human Environment. Proceedings of a Joint Symposium. IARC scientific publication no. 53. Lyon, France: International Agency for Research on Cancer; 1984. pp. 487-495

[63] Grandjean P. Human exposure to nickel. In: Sunderman FW Jr, editor. Nickel in the Human Environment. Proceedings of a Joint Symposium. IARC scientific publication no. 53. Lyon, France: International Agency for Research on Cancer; 1984. pp. 469-485

[64] Sunderman FW Jr, Oskarsson A. Nickel. In: Merian E, editor. Metals and their Compounds in the Environment. New York: VCH Verlagsgesellschaft; 1991. pp. 1101-1126

[65] Nielsen NH, Menné T, Kristiansen J, Christensen JM, Borg L, Poulsen LK. Effects of repeated skin exposure to low nickel concentrations: A model for allergic contact dermatitis to nickel on the hands. The British Journal of Dermatology. 1999;**141**:676-682

[66] Patriarca M, Lyon TD, Fell GS. Nickel metabolism in humans investigated with an oral stable isotope. The American Journal of Clinical Nutrition. 1997;**66**:616-621

[67] Sunderman FW Jr. Mechanisms of nickel carcinogenesis. Scandinavian Journal of Work, Environment & Health. 1989;**15**:1-12

[68] Fullerton A, Andersen JR, Hoelgaard A, Menné T. Permeation of nickel salts through human skin in vitro. Contact Dermatitis. 1986;**15**:173-177

[69] Norgaard O. Investigation with radioactive Ni-57 into the resorption of nickel through the skin in normal and in

nickelhypersensitive persons. Acta Dermato-Venereologica. 1955;**35**:111-117

[70] Bernacki EJ, Parsons GE, Sunderman FW Jr. Investigation of exposure to nickel and lung cancer mortality. Annals of Clinical and Laboratory Science. 1978; **8**:190-194

[71] Elias Z, Mur JM, Pierre F, Gilgenkrantz S, Schneider O, Baruthio F, et al. Chromosome aberrations in peripheral blood lymphocytes of welders and characterization of their exposure by biological samples analysis. Journal of Occupational Medicine. 1989;**31**: 477-483

[72] Angerer J, Lehnert G. Occupational chronic exposure to metals. II: Nickel exposure of stainless steel welders-biological monitoring. International Archives of Occupational and Environmental Health. 1990;**62**:7-10

[73] Sunderman FW Jr, Hopfer SM, Sweeney KR, Marcus AH, Most BM, Creason J. Nickel absorption and kinetics in human volunteers. Proceedings of the Society for Experimental Biology and Medicine. 1989;**191**:5-11

[74] Cangul H, Broday L, Salnikow K, Sutherland J, Peng W, Zhang Q, Poltaratsky V, et al. Molecular mechanisms of nickel carcinogenesis. Toxicology Letters. 2002;**127**:69-75

[75] Heck JD, Costa M. Surface reduction of amorphous nis particles potentiates their phagocytosis and subsequent induction of morphological transformation in Syrian hamster embryo cells. Cancer Letters. 1982;**15**: 19-26

[76] Glennon JD, Sarkar B. Nickel(ii) transport in human blood serum: Studies of nickel(ii)-binding human albumin and to native-sequence peptide, and ternary complex formation with l-histidine. The Biochemical Journal. 1982; **203**:15-23

[77] Nielsen JL, Poulsen OM, Abildtrup A. Studies of serum protein complexes with nickel using crossed immunoelectrophoresis. Electrophoresis. 1994;**15**:666-671

[78] Valko M, Morris H, Cronin MTD. Metals, toxicity and oxidative stress. Current Medicinal Chemistry. 2005;**12**: 1161-1208

[79] Oller AR, Costa M, Oberdörster G. Carcinogenicity assessment of selected nickel compounds. Toxicology and Applied Pharmacology. 1997;**143**: 152-166

[80] Mcgregor DB, Baan RA, Partensky C, Rice JM, Wilbourn JD. Evaluation of the carcinogenic risks to humans associated with surgical implants and other foreign bodies – A report of an iarc monographs programme meeting. European Journal of Cancer. 2000;**36**:307-313

[81] WHO Regional Office for Europe. Chapter 6.10. In: Nickel Air Quality Guidelines. Second ed. Copenhagen, Denmark: WHO Regional Office for Europe; 2000

[82] Agency for Toxic Substances and Disease Registry. Toxicological Profile for Chromium. 2000. Available from: http://www.atsdr.cdc.gov/toprofiles/tp7.html

[83] Aitio A, Jarvisalo J, et al. Urinary excretion of chromium as an indicator of exposure to trivalent chromium sulphate in leather tanning. International Archives of Occupational & Environmental Health. 1984;**54**(3): 241-249

[84] Foa V, Riboldi L, et al. Effects derived from long-term low-level chromium exposure in ferro-alloy metallurgy. Study of absorption and renal function in workers. Science of the Total Environment. 1988;**71**(3):389-400

[85] Dayan AD, Paine AJ. Mechanisms of chromium toxicity, carcinogenicity and allergenicity: Review of the literature from 1985 to 2000. Human & Experimental Toxicology. 2001;**20**(9): 439-451

[86] Cohen MD, Kargacin B, et al. Mechanisms of chromium carcinogenicity and toxicity. Critical Reviews in Toxicology. 1993;**23**(3): 255-281

[87] Baranowska-Dutkiewicz B. Absorption of hexavalent chromium by skin in man. Archives of Toxicology. 1981;**47**(1):47-50

[88] EPA. Toxicological review of trivalent chromium. CAS No. 16065-83-1. In: Support of Summary Information on the Integrated Risk Information System (IRIS). Washington, D.C.: U.S. Environmental Protection Agency; 1998

[89] Kiilunen M, Kivisto H, et al. Exceptional pharmacokinetics of trivalent chromium during occupational exposure to chromium lignosulfonate dust. Scandinavian Journal of Work, Environment & Health. 1983;**9**(3): 265-271

[90] Novey HS, Habib M, et al. Asthma and IgE antibodies induced by chromium and nickel salts. Journal of Allergy & Clinical Immunology. 1983; **72**(4):407-412

[91] Deng JF, Fleeger AK, et al. An outbreak of chromium ulcer in a manufacturing plant. Veterinary & Human Toxicology. 1990;**32**(2):142-146

[92] Geller R. Chromium. In: Sullivan JB Jr, Krieger GR, editors. Clinical Environmental Health and Toxic Exposures. 2nd ed. Philadelphia, PA: Lippincott Williams & Wilkins; 2001

[93] Sharma BK, Singhal PC, et al. Intravascular haemolysis and acute renal failure following potassium dichromate poisoning. Postgraduate Medical Journal. 1978;**54**(632):414-415

[94] Agency for Toxic Substances and Disease Registry. Toxicological Profile for Cobalt. 2000. Available from: http://www.atsdr.cdc.gov/toprofiles/tp7.html.

[95] Smith IC, Carson BL. Trace Metals in the Environment. Ann Arbor, MI: Ann Arbor Science Publishers; 1981

[96] Kreyling WG, Godleski JJ, Kariya ST, et al. In vitro dissolution of uniform cobalt oxide particles by human and canine alveolar macrophages. American Journal of Respiratory Cell and Molecular Biology. 1990;**2**:413-422

[97] Smith RJ. I. the effect of cobalt on hydrolase activity in kidney and plasma and its relationship to erythropoietin production. II. Structure activity relationships of several protein and polypeptide potentiators of bradykinin action on rat uterus. Dissertation Abstracts International B. 1972;**32**(10): 6132

[98] Sorbie J, Olatunbosun D, Corbett WEN, et al. Cobalt excretion test for the assessment of body iron stores. Canadian Medical Association Journal. 1971;**104**(9):777-782

[99] Vouk VB. General chemistry of metals. In: Friberg L, Nordberg GF, Vouk VB, editors. Handbook on the Toxicology of Metals. 2nd ed. New York, NY: Elsevier Science Publishers; 1986. pp. 33-34

[100] Domingo JL. Cobalt in the environment and its toxicological implications. Reviews of Environmental Contamination and Toxicology. 1989; **108**:105-132

[101] Apostoli P, Porru S, Alessio L. Urinary cobalt excretion in short time occupational exposure to cobalt powders. Science of the Total Environment. 1994;**150**:129-132

[102] Mosconi G, Bacis M, Vitali MT, et al. Cobalt excretion in urine: Results of a study on workers producing diamond grinding tools and on a control group. Science of the Total Environment. 1994b;**150**:133-139

[103] Beleznay E, Osvay M. Long-term clearance of accidentally inhaled 60Co aerosols in humans. Health Physics. 1994;**66**:392-399

[104] Bailey MR, Kreyling WG, Andre S, et al. An interspecies comparison of the lung clearance of inhaled monodisperse cobalt oxide particles- part 1: Objectives and summary of results. Journal of Aerosol Science. 1989;**20**(2):169-188

[105] Newton D, Rundo J. The long term retention of inhaled cobalt-60. Health Physics. 1971;**21**(3):377-384

[106] Foster PP, Pearman I, Ramsden D. An interspecies comparison of the lung clearance of inhaled monodisperse cobalt oxide particles- part II: Lung clearance of inhaled cobalt oxide in man. Journal of Aerosol Science. 1989;**20**(2):189-204

[107] Scansetti G, Botta GC, Spinelli P, et al. Absorption and excretion of cobalt in the hard metal industry. Science of the Total Environment. 1994;**150**:141-144

[108] Agency for Toxic Substances and Disease Registry. Toxicological Profile for Molybdenum. 2000. Available from: http://www.atsdr.cdc.gov/toprofiles/tp7.html.

[109] NAS. Molybdenum. In: Dietary Reference Intakes for Vitamin a, Vitamin K, Arsenic, Boron, Chromium, Copper, Iodine, Iron, Manganese, Molybdenum, Nickel, Silicon, Vanadium, and Zinc. Washington, DC: National Academies Press; 2001. pp. 420-439

[110] EPA. 1979. Human health effects of molybdenum in drinking water. U.S. Environmental Protection Agency. EPA600179006. PB292755. Available from: http://nepis.epa.gov/Exe/ZyPURL.cgi?Dockey=2000Z0FV.txt [Accessed: October 2, 2015]

[111] Barceloux DG. Molybdenum. Journal of Toxicology. Clinical Toxicology. 1999;**37**(2):231-237

[112] Bailey MR, Ansoborlo E, Guilmette RA, et al. Updating the ICRP human respiratory tract model. Radiation Protection Dosimetry. 2007; **127**(1–4):31-34

[113] ICRP. Molybdenum. International commission on radiological protection. Annals of the ICRP. 1994;**23**(3–4):45-47

[114] Nakanishi Y, Iida S, Ueoka-Nakanishi H, et al. Exploring dynamics of molybdate in living animal cells by a genetically encoded FRET nanosensor. PLoS One. 2013;**8**(3):e58175. DOI: 10.1371/journal.pone.0058175

[115] Mendel RR, Kruse T. Cell biology of molybdenum in plants and humans. Biochimica et Biophysica Acta. 2012; **1823**(9):1568-1579. DOI: 10.1016/j.bbamcr.2012.02.007

[116] Schwarz G, Mendel RR, Ribbe MW. Molybdenum cofactors, enzymes and pathways. Nature. 2009;**460**:839-847

[117] Nederbragt H. The influence of molybdenum on the copper metabolism of the rat at different Cu levels of the diet. The British Journal of Nutrition. 1980;**43**(2):329-338

[118] Nederbragt H. Changes in the distribution of copper and molybdenum after Mo administration and subsequent additional oral or intraperitoneal Cu administration to rats. The British Journal of Nutrition. 1982;**48**(2):353-364

[119] Giussani A. A recycling systemic model for the biokinetics of molybdenum radionuclides. Science of the Total Environment. 2008;**404**(1): 44-55. DOI: 10.1016/j.scitotenv.2008.06.019

[120] Novotny JA, Turnlund JR. Molybdenum intake influences molybdenum kinetics in men. The Journal of Nutrition. 2007;**137**(1):37-42

[121] Brewer GJ, Dick RD, Grover DK, et al. Treatment of metastatic cancer with tetrathiomolybdate, an anticopper, antiangiogenic agent: Phase I study. Clinical Cancer Research. 2000;**6**(1): 1-10

[122] Deosthale YG, Gopalan C. The effect of molybdenum levels in sorghum (Sorghum vulgare Pers.) on uric acid and copper excretion in man. The British Journal of Nutrition. 1974;**31**(3):351-355

[123] Turnlund JR, Keyes WR. Dietary molybdenum. Effect on copper absorption, excretion, and status in young men. In: Trace Elements in Man and Animals. New York, NY: Plenum Publishers; 2000. pp. 951-953

[124] Bhaskar V, Reddy S. Biodegradation of nickel and chromium from space maintainers: An in vitro study. Journal of Indian Society of Pedodontics Preventive Dentistry. 2010;**28**:6-12

[125] Keinan D, Mass E, Zilberman U. Absorption of nickel, chromium, and iron by the root surface of primary molars covered with stainless steel crowns. International Journal of Dentistry. 2010;**2010**:326124 4 pages

[126] Kodaira H, Ohno K, Fukase N, Kuroda M, Adachi S, Kikuchi M, et al. Release and systemic accumulation of heavy metals frompreformed crowns used in restoration of primary teeth. Journal of Oral Science. 2013;**55**(2): 161-165

[127] Kulkarni P, Agrawal S, Bansal A, Jain A, Tiwari U, Anand A. Assessment of nickel release from various dental appliances used routinely in pediatric dentistry. Indian Journal of Dentistry. 2016;**7**:81-85

[128] Basir L, Shamsaei M, Ziaei SA. Evaluation of nickel releasing from stainless steel crowns regarding to "trimming": An in vitro study. Journal of Indian Society of Pedodontics and Preventive Dentistry. 2018;**36**:58-64